Electroconvulsive Therapy in America

W0234929

Electroconvulsive therapy is widely demonized or idealized. Some detractors consider its very use to be a human rights violation, while some promoters depict it as a miracle, the "penicillin of psychiatry." This book traces the American history of one of the most controversial procedures in medicine, and seeks to provide an explanation of *why* ECT has been so controversial, juxtaposing evidence from clinical science, personal memoir, and popular culture. Contextualizing the controversies about ECT, instead of simply engaging in them, makes the history of ECT more richly revealing of wider changes in culture and medicine. It shows that the application of electricity to the brain to treat illness is not only a physiological event, but also one embedded in culturally patterned beliefs about the human body, the meaning of sickness, and medical authority.

Jonathan Sadowsky is the Theodore J. Castele Professor of Medical History at Case Western Reserve University.

Routledge Studies in Cultural History

For a full list of titles in this series, please visit www.routledge.com

Electroconvulsive Therapy in America

The Anatomy of a Medical Controversy

Jonathan Sadowsky

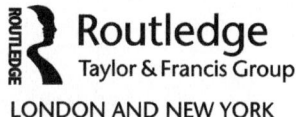

Routledge
Taylor & Francis Group

LONDON AND NEW YORK

First published 2017 by Routledge

2 Park Square, Milton Park, Abingdon, Oxfordshire OX14 4RN

52 Vanderbilt Avenue, New York, NY 10017

Routledge is an imprint of the Taylor & Francis Group, an informa business

First issued in paperback 2019

Library of Congress Cataloging in Publication Data
Names: Sadowsky, Jonathan, author.
Title: Electroconvulsive therapy in America : the anatomy of a medical controversy / by Jonathan Sadowsky.
Description: New York : Routledge, 2017. | Series: Routledge studies in cultural history ; 49 | Includes bibliographical references and index.
Identifiers: LCCN 2016030702 (print) | LCCN 2016032120 (ebook) | ISBN 9781138696969 (hbk : alk. paper) | ISBN 9781315522852 (ebk) | ISBN 9781315522852
Subjects: LCSH: Electroconvulsive therapy—United States—History.
Classification: LCC RC485 .S23 2017 (print) | LCC RC485 (ebook) | DDC 616.89/122—dc23
LC record available at https://lccn.loc.gov/2016030702

ISBN: 978-1-138-69696-9 (hbk)
ISBN: 978-0-367-26406-2 (pbk)

Typeset in Sabon
by Apex CoVantage, LLC

For My Parents

Contents

Acknowledgments

My family, most of all, of course. My parents encouraged love of learning and commitment to reason from my infancy, and have been sounding boards for my ideas all through adulthood. My mother developed Alzheimer's disease midway through the work of this project, so I have been grappling with problems of memory in my scholarly work and in my personal life. She is no longer at a point where she can appreciate this book; she would have been so happy to see it. My father has been a rock of support for her throughout. He has been the same for me my whole life. Thanks also to my brother Richard, and my sister Nina, great friends and supports. Both of my children, Ivan and Julia, were born while I was working on this book, and I have been so lucky to have such sweet, funny, creative kids. Finally, of course, Laura. I knew I wanted to marry her within a few weeks of meeting her 25 years ago. Whatever flaws there may be to this book, that choice alone redeems my judgment.

I have to single out three CWRU colleagues for exceptional support. Alan Rocke has been my professional mentor for a quarter of a century. He has read every word of peer-reviewed writing I have ever submitted, and he has always found time to discuss any research, teaching, or university governance issue I wanted. Eileen Anderson-Fye has been a true friend, and a bit of an intellectual twin. I've rarely met another scholar who thought about things so much the way I do. Ted Steinberg has been challenging me for two decades to think as deeply as possibly about the ultimate ends of historiography. We don't always come to the same answers, but mine are better for having grappled with his. Plus, I sometimes feel he would walk through the gates of Hades for me if I asked him to.

Not all academic departments are environments of mutual support, and I know I am lucky to be in one that is. I would especially like to thank Renee Sentilles, Peter Shulman, and Gillian Weiss for their stimulation and support; Peter read and commented on the entire manuscript. Other CWRU colleagues whose support and intellect this book has benefited from are Francesca Brittan, Jim Edmonson, Kim Emmons, Chris Flint, Kenny Fountain, Laura Hengehold, Marixa Lasso, and Athena Vrettos.

I have also profited from conversations with colleagues elsewhere, including Linda Andre, Joel Braslow, John Burnham, David William Cohen, Deborah Doroshow, Jacalyn Duffin, Marta Elliott, Max Fink, Matt Gambino, Bert Hansen, Laura Hirshbein, Richard Keller, Charles Kellner, Barron Lerner, Marvin Lipkowitz, Julie Livingston, Emily Martin, Karen Maschke, Doug McLaughlin, George Makari, Mical Raz, Geoffrey Reaume, Susan Reverby, Naomi Rogers, David Rothman, Harold Sackeim, Andrea Tone, and John Harley Warner.

I am of course especially grateful to those colleagues who read all or part of the manuscript at some point: Jesse Ballenger, Stephen Casper, Jennifer Fishman, Janet Golden, Jenell Johnson, Nick King, Beth Linker, Liz Lunbeck, and Hans Pols.

The work profited from presentations I gave at a number of venues, including the Richardson Seminar in the History of Psychiatry at Cornell/ Weill, the Institute for the History of the Medicine at the Johns Hopkins University, the New York Academy of Medicine, the History Department at Oberlin College, the Department of the History of Medicine at the University of Wisconsin, Madison, the Science and Technology Studies Program at the University of Michigan, the History of Medicine Department at the University of Minnesota, the Department of the History of Medicine at Yale University, the History Department at Washington University in St. Louis, the Center for the History of Psychology at the University of Akron, and the Cleveland Psychoanalytic Center. I am grateful for the invitations to present, and for the audience commentary that followed in each instance.

I have had several talented research assistants helping me over the course of the project: Geoff Zylstra, the late Judi Northwood, and Katie Schroeder. Beth Salem, in particular, has been a skilled and dedicated partner for years.

I would also like to thank two graduate students, Katie Schaub and Kristi Ninneman, who provided me with thoughtful criticism on some of the chapters.

Thanks also to those librarians and archivists who provided assistance: Elsie Finley, Andrew Harrison, Andrew Dorchak, Diane Richardson, Lisa Peters, and Bill Claspy.

The project received financial support from a Senior Faculty research grant from the Ohio Board of Regents, and a grant from the Howard Foundation.

Introduction

Hope or Horror?

> *"Why, after the 'amazingly short' three or so shock treatments did I rocket uphill? Why did I feel I needed to be punished, to punish myself."*
> —Sylvia Plath[1]

As one of the most iconic public figures associated with mental illness, Sylvia Plath's story is well known in some ways. But I want to begin with her because of the ways it is not. Plath made her experience with electroconvulsive therapy a central motif in both her fiction and her poetry. In *The Bell Jar*, Plath's protagonist Esther Greenwood—often read as Plath's alter ego—describes the treatment like this:

> Then something bent down and took hold of me and shook me like the end of the world. Whee-eeee-ee, it shrilled, through an air crackling with blue light, and with each flash a great jolt drubbed me till I thought my bones would break and the sap would fly out of me like a split plant.
> I wondered what terrible thing it was that I had done.[2]

This passage was cited by historian Roy Porter to show that "twentieth-century [psychiatric] patients have been more vocal about the horrors of involuntary ECT than any other issue."[3]

In fact, neither Greenwood's nor Plath's ECT was involuntary. Greenwood, like her creator Plath, agreed to ECT in the hopes of reducing her acute suffering. And in *The Bell Jar*, it led to remission of painful symptoms, as it did in Plath's life. Plath's account is also complicated by a record of her literary ambitions in her journals. She was driven to reach a large audience; noting that there was a growing popularity for asylum literature, she wrote to herself, "I *must* write one about a college girl suicide . . . and a story, a novel even. Must get out SNAKE PIT."[4] But if Plath's representation is not a straightforward condemnation of ECT, it cannot be reduced to sensationalism and opportunism, either. Greenwood feared ECT, as Plath herself did.

Plath's own story might best be regarded as a tale of two ECTs. After spiraling down to severe depression while a student at Smith College, she had several traumatizing ECT treatments in 1953 at Valley Head Hospital in Massachusetts. In a later hospitalization at McLean Psychiatric Hospital outside of Boston, however, a doctor persuaded an understandably reluctant Plath to try again, and in this case, ECT treatments made her feel much better. Hence the quote in her journal, "Why, after the 'amazingly short' three or so shock treatments did I rocket uphill? Why did I feel I needed to be punished, to punish myself."[5] This reflection contains both an acknowledgment of therapeutic power, and an assumption that that power is due to a punitive effect.

Plath's experience captures a duality that runs through the history of ECT: a capacity to heal and help, and a power to harm and horrify. This duality is in many ways *the* story of the history of ECT. Yet it has been oddly avoided in most historical treatments.[6] It is the main theme in what follows here.

The Dynamics of a Controversy

Electroconvulsive therapy is the application of electricity to the body in order to induce seizures, and ultimately relieve symptoms of major mental illnesses, such as severe and chronic depression. Depictions of it are perhaps the most divided in medicine. Commonly known to laypeople as "shock treatment," it is thought by many to be an abandoned medical practice, like lobotomy, although a revival of the practice has been underway for about three decades—nearly a generation now. This revival has received some media attention, and this attention often contains assurances that the therapy is not as frightening as many believe. Yet many continue to fear ECT—it is the cultural icon for psychiatric abuse, and some former patients and their allies continue to campaign against its use. Many doctors tout it as the most effective treatment in psychiatry, a safe and humane option that provides powerful relief from the ravages of serious affective disorder, and they have the testimony of many grateful patients to support them. Reading different accounts of the therapy can feel like moving between alternate realities.

In the nation's collective memory, ECT often appears as a remnant, a vestigial limb of medicine. Many twentieth-century medical developments fostered deep, and sometimes blind, faith in medical progress, a faith that has never been well extended to ECT. Public fears have been dramatized in numerous novels and films, including the most influential rendering in *One Flew Over the Cuckoo's Nest,* which remains the most vivid cultural association for prospective patients. ECT has become a symbol not only for coerciveness in psychiatry, but for arbitrary authority generally, even as many psychiatrists, and many patients, view ECT as a life-saving technology.

It may be controversial even to *call* ECT controversial. In *Psychiatric Times,* two prominent practitioners, Charles Kellner and Max Fink, co-authored an article in which they asserted that it was factually wrong to describe ECT as controversial.[7] Several months later, Kellner published an article in the very same publication in which he described ECT as the "second most controversial procedure in medicine," the first being abortion. Rather than reflecting an inconsistency on Kellner's part, this discrepancy probably represents an ambiguity over what it means to call ECT controversial. In the first article they meant that the overwhelming scientific support should mean that ECT should not be controversial. In the second case Kellner acknowledged that, like it or not, many people do not acknowledge the validity of the scientific support.[8] Kellner's comparison with abortion is also worth attention. Abortion is much more common, garners much more public attention, is much more salient in our political culture. But one of the reasons abortion is so controversial is that it reflects fundamental disagreements over wider issues, such as normative human sexuality, and the very definition of a person. As I will show, the controversies over ECT also reflect deeper conflicts. Partly these conflicts are medical: what kind of psychiatry should we have? But they are also conflicts over very deeply held and often implicit ethical and metaphysical assumptions. They, too, may even reflect disagreements over what a person is.

Controversy is also reflected in the various names given to this treatment. The most commonly recognized colloquial terms are "shock treatment" and "shock therapy," and although these names are sometimes used for convenience even by people who are supporters, they inevitably carry some taint of horror, extremity, or abuse. Like many medical terms, these have migrated into other domains—primarily economics, where they refer to rapidly administered government austerity programs.[9] Although adopted by austerity advocates to help justify their practices, the term deliberately conveys both short-term pain that needs to be endured for future healing, as well as extreme measures needed because of desperate circumstances. The clinical term "electroconvulsive therapy" is preferred by practitioners, partly because it is less threatening, and partly because it is precise in terms of clinical rationale: ECT is therapy that utilizes electricity to induce convulsions.[10] This being the official medical name for the therapy, it will be the term I use in this book.

The small historiography of ECT has so far reproduced the controversy more than it has explained it. Book-length treatments include Carole Warren and Timothy Kneeland's *Pushbutton Psychiatry* and Edward Shorter and David Healy's 2007 *Shock Therapy*.[11] Kneeland and Warren depict ECT as a tool of social control, used by psychiatry to enforce gender and sexual conformity. There is no discussion of any possible clinical efficacy, a subject they explicitly disavow competence to make judgments about. Shorter and Healy, by contrast, depict ECT as virtually unalloyed medical progress, a heroic advance that has been unfairly stigmatized.

My primary purpose is not to pull the conversation into a middle ground, but rather to reach a greater understanding of why it became so polarized to begin with. Explaining the controversy is not important because controversy should be defused, or because balance is always a supreme good. ECT matters in part because the history of its controversy, if grounded in both medical and cultural history, has much more to tell us about our changing medical cultures, and ultimately the historically formed nature of self and body.

What Is ECT? Why Is There ECT?

The idea of inducing convulsions by running electricity through the brain is more than a little counter-intuitive. It seems to many people not only weird, but possibly inherently violent. Although more detail on its origin will come in Chapter One, it is worth pausing now to ask, why did people start doing this in the first place?

Attempts to use electricity for therapy date to antiquity.[12] In the eighteenth century, Swedish researchers found it useful in some cases of paralysis and epilepsy, and in Britain, clinicians reported success applying electricity to the body for "hysterical" and "nervous" conditions. Attempts specifically to induce convulsions, by electricity or other means, were also employed for mental illness at that time.[13] Over the course of the nineteenth century, there were numerous and varied attempts to apply electricity to human bodies for therapeutic purposes, including psychiatric ones. Not all of these were intended to induce convulsions, though.

The development of ECT derives most directly from the belief of some twentieth-century psychiatrists and neurologists that there might be an inverse correlation between schizophrenia and epilepsy, which were thought rarely to appear in the same person. Hungarian neuropathologist Ladislas von Meduna noticed that glia cells in schizophrenic patients appeared very different from those in epileptic patients. In the early 1930s, he began to use the chemical Metrazol to induce convulsions in psychotic patients.[14]

According to most accounts, Metrazol, or chemical convulsive therapy, was an effective but scary treatment. Virtually all contemporaries who attested to its efficacy remarked on the feeling of terror patients would feel at the beginning of a treatment, particularly if they had already had one. This description is from a psychiatric textbook written by doctors who favored its use, who considered ECT an in improvement, but not so great a one as to render the others obsolete:[15]

> One of the greatest drawbacks to pharmacologic convulsive therapy is the fear the patient experiences between injection and onset of convulsion. The patient does not lose consciousness as long as no convulsion takes place. In the interval between injection and convulsion he has what is described as a feeling of impending death and sudden annihilation.[16]

A few years after Meduna reported success with chemical convulsive therapy, Italian psychiatrists Ugo Cerletti and Lucio Bini developed ECT in the hopes of finding an easier and safer way to induce convulsions.[17] It is one of the ironies of ECT's history that it was developed in an attempt to make convulsive therapy less scary and more humane, and it then became a cultural symbol for medical terror.

In modern usage, a patient who receives ECT is most usually one who has suffered from a severe mood disorder for some time without improvement from other treatments, or one who has benefited from the treatment in the past.[18] The patient is given anesthesia to prevent pain from the treatment and muscle relaxants to prevent injury from the seizures; this is known as "modified" ECT, differentiating it from the cruder applications originally developed. Consent is required in the vast majority of cases. Whether the information typically provided is adequate is one of the subjects of controversy. Patients are often told that there will be short-term memory loss, mostly of events near the treatment, and that the memories will typically return. The risk of permanent memory loss is often described as minimal, and critics claim this understates the risk. I look at this problem in detail in Chapter Six.

ECT, Efficacy, and the History of Therapeutics

While working on this project, I have often been asked, does ECT work? This is a fair question, and not one historians should dodge. The quick answer is yes, ECT works, in a limited sense that its proponents claim, and have claimed since it was invented: it provides quick, although not necessarily lasting, relief from the symptoms of severe mental illness. This, in fact, has not been the subject of much controversy. There has been much more dispute over whether it has costs that are unacceptable.

A few medical historians have, in recent years, scrutinized the question of efficacy—that is, does a treatment work? Is the very meaning of a treatment working historically variable? In a well-known essay, Charles Rosenberg lamented how little attention historians of medicine had paid to the subject of therapeutics—meaning, the history of medical procedures in practice, as distinct from the history of medical ideas and knowledge.[19] Rosenberg thought that historians had avoided the subject because it raised a question that many found "embarrassing," namely the problem of efficacy. How could historians square their desire to respect past therapies with the knowledge that those practices were, in hindsight, primitive or misguided? Rosenberg began with a plea for a respectful attention to past therapeutic practices, combined with an anthropological understanding that they "worked," in their context—that is, they worked in a social, not an objective, medical sense. Rosenberg's article raised some important questions, but started with a misreading of what it means to think "anthropologically" about a medical treatment. For Rosenberg, if a treatment was not part of the repertoire of modern biomedicine, an anthropologist might try to imagine why it *seemed* to work, even though we know it did not. The anthropological literature on efficacy, however, mostly takes the opposite tack—it seeks to understand how it is that practices outside of biomedicine do, in fact, work.[20]

Though Rosenberg's article was influential, discussions of it sometimes omit his conclusion—that while judging discarded therapies in context is a worthy historical exercise, in the end we need to recognize the reality of medical progress, the superiority of later therapeutics. Obsolete treatments, in this view, deserve enough respect that we should understand how they were *perceived* to work, but we should recognize when they have been surpassed by scientifically better ones. John Harley Warner took the problem a step further, emphasizing that the meaning of what it is to say a treatment "works" changes historically.[21] Therapeutics of the early nineteenth century saw disease as an overstimulated aberration from a natural state. Practices such as bloodletting worked because the depletion allowed a return to the natural state, and provided some sense of relief to patients by inducing dramatic and undeniable physiological changes. This provoked Warner (particularly in the preface to the second edition) to raise some probing questions about the status of later scientific medicine and ultimately about medical progress. If each system of therapeutics works according to its own standards, can we really say that any one is better than another? Any concessions Warner made to therapeutic relativism stopped at the border of his own body, though. He conceded that he planned, personally, on following the therapeutic regimens of the late twentieth century, on the grounds that he was invested in the therapeutics of his own era. The limits to my own relativism may be stricter. Medical progress may not be linear or teleological, but I do think it is possible, and I will be making a cautious argument that we do have a better somatic psychiatry now than we had a century ago.

Jack Pressman's history of lobotomy advanced the historical study of efficacy by using the example of this reviled treatment as a challenge to images of the march of medical progress. Pressman rendered those images a bit ironically:

> Typically, the explanation of how a new treatment achieved widespread acceptance by the medical profession reduces to this: it was effective, spectacularly and undeniably so. Diphtheria antitoxin saved a young girl's life on Christmas Eve, 1895; penicillin prevented countless thousands of gangrene-related amputations during the Second World War; and so on. The usual parade of such examples reinforces belief in the supposition that the life course of a medical innovation is determined mostly by the treatment's inherent soundness. Procedures that work, fly and are assured of their place in the medical record; those that do not, crash and appropriately find only oblivion. The true value of any particular therapy is thus assumed to be a quality that is both immediate and yet transcendent, equally visible across the decades.[22]

Lobotomy, it would seem, had fallen the way of oblivion. By this logic, one might assume it did not work. Following Rosenberg, Pressman seeks to depose such a progress narrative in favor of a sensitive understanding of why a "drastic" (his word) procedure was deemed effective.[23] Given how steeped American culture and medical historiography had once been in unreflective celebrations of medical progress, this kind of challenge is understandable. He was also attempting to make comprehensible a medical practice that had, with the passage of time, come to seem incomprehensible.

Pressman's rendering of lobotomy, though, is more a story of progress than he allows. Lobotomy was adopted, he shows, because although it did not cure a specific disease, it provided some relief to suffering patients and their families. The costs of this relief were not immediately apparent. Lobotomy did, then, mark progress in a context where the chronically mentally ill could be offered little else. As the costs in cognitive decline associated with lobotomy became more apparent, and safer alternatives became available in the form of antipsychotic medications, it was phased out. Psychosurgery rose because of the evidence of effectiveness, and declined because of the evidence for better treatments. This is how progress in clinical science is supposed to work.

In his history of somatic treatments for mental illness in the early twentieth century, Braslow distinguishes between efficacy and effectiveness.[24] Effectiveness refers to everyday clinical performance, the routine observation that people seem to get better. Efficacy, by contrast, is performance in controlled tests—or, in other words, a treatment is scientifically proven to work by our current standards. The distinction is helpful for understanding discarded therapies in their context. It is not as helpful for understanding ECT, though, because unlike the other therapies Braslow studies, ECT has shown good results in controlled trials.

Much of the historiography of therapeutic efficacy so far has in fact focused on discarded treatments—those that have, in the view of biomedical science, been rendered obsolete. These are the ones that threaten the embarrassment that worried Rosenberg. If a treatment is still used and regarded as scientifically sound, we appear to be absolved of the labor of anthropologically understanding why people once thought it worked—although contemporary practices may be probed by actual anthropologists, who have provocatively shown ritualistic or other extra-scientific factors in belief in a medical procedure.[25] Historians studying extant therapies have tended to treat their efficacy as a given; penicillin, the polio vaccine, and aspirin, for example, have received histories where the physiological efficacy of the treatment is an integral part of the meaning of the story of success.[26] Historicizing therapies still in use is possible—I intend to do it in what follows—but it poses a different set of challenges, and responsibilities, from historicizing discarded ones.

I have occasionally been urged, by very smart colleagues, to evade judgments about clinical efficacy altogether. This, some historians say, is simply not our job. We should stick to tracing the histories of what people have said about it, including what they—patients, clinicians, and other observers—*have said* about whether it works. I understand this impulse, but disagree with it. I wonder whether those who offer this advice have a lingering suspicion of ECT, an assumption that it should not, cannot work. Allow me a reduction to the absurd: would a historian of technology writing about the history of airplanes be urged to "bracket" the question of whether they actually fly, in favor of a history of "representations of flying efficacy"? There are important critical questions to be asked about the history of aviation, as there are with any technology, but asking whether planes fly is not one of them. Saying that ECT works is indeed, of course, more complicated. It has been used in different ways at different times, and efficacy in the treatment of mental illness inevitably has complex meanings. These problems are taken seriously in what follows. But the comparison underscores a serious point: a historian of penicillin, or chemotherapy for cancer, is not typically advised, by any but the most zealous social constructionist, to bracket the question of whether these treatments work.

And bracketing the question has costs. It is the approach Kneeland and Warren take. They decline to answer the question of whether ECT works, saying that they are historians, not clinicians, and are therefore qualified only to look at what ECT means. But what if an important part of the story is that for many people suffering from serious illness, its meaning is exactly that it works? There is also a strange irony to this modesty, because they feel competent to assess that ECT is in fact effective—as a means of social control. This selective modesty is mirrored in Shorter and Healy's celebratory account of ECT. They (both historians, although Healy is also a psychiatrist) most definitely assert competence to say ECT works. That is in fact the main point of their book. But they say historical methods are poor tools for making judgments on the vexed question of the extent to which ECT causes memory loss.[27] I argue, especially in Chapter Six, that it is indeed challenging to make definitive judgments about how common permanent memory losses are, but careful historical attention to both the clinical science and the narrative evidence available should make us very hesitant to conclude that it is rare. Consequently, any assessment of ECT's efficacy requires a deeper assessment of its possible costs.

Pressman argued that the question "does it work?" leads to arid interpretation because it is not a historical question. It may not be the most historical question we can ask. But it is also not a question that can be left out of clinical history, especially the history of a controversial procedure. ECT's continued use makes it a pressing question. If it does not work, its practitioners are either deluded or perverse, and its patients are getting electricity passed through their brain for no good reason.

There are good reasons to believe that ECT works in contemporary psychiatry in the way psychiatrists say it works—as a means of relieving symptoms of serious mental illnesses, especially affective disorders, such as major depression. One is the simple, experience-based kind of working knowledge that doctors have used since the beginnings of medicine: they see the improvement in their patients. The second is more reflective of contemporary scientific norms, reflecting the use of a kind of knowledge that became especially common in medicine after World War II: the randomized clinical trial (RCT).[28] My own tendencies toward historical relativism are tempered by respect for the RCT as a powerful epistemological tool, for all its imperfections. While all knowledge has a social basis, and we should always be alert to the ways science might be shaped by subjective factors, the RCT was an important advance in the production of medical knowledge, because it carefully compares groups of patients who receive a treatment with groups who do not. RCTs can show when a treatment is benefiting a greater number of patients than might have gotten better through a placebo effect, or simply through spontaneous remission.

Controlled studies of ECT generally show high rates of symptom relief.[29] In fact some clinical scientists regard the evidence for its efficacy to be "among the most robust for any medical treatment."[30] These studies include comparisons with "sham" or fake ECT as controls, although controlled studies of ECT pose practical and ethical challenges.[31] Efficacy in these studies is not cure, in the sense of providing permanent or lifelong freedom from the illness following one course of treatment. Some patients may obtain this, but this is not what the clinicians are offering. Cure in this sense remains hard to come by for severe mental illness treated by any means, so efficacy is judged by symptom relief. The efficacy rates reported for ECT are often in the range of 80–90%, although lower, in the range of 50–60%, for depression that has been resistant to treatment by medication.[32] These are the results of a large number of studies, done over the course of many years. Some critics of clinical trials rightly complain of a publication bias in favor of positive results—researchers have more to gain by publishing positive results, and journals prefer to publish positive results.[33] But even if this complaint is valid, it would not explain why ECT would have higher success rates than antidepressant medications in the studies.

Perhaps the most important historical point to make about ECT and efficacy is that it has been perceived as effective both in the era prior to widespread RCTs and in the present. Among psychiatrists, it has been rare to find practitioners who do not think ECT works, although there are those who oppose it because they regard it as unsafe. But if psychiatrists of all kinds, and in all eras, said it worked and patients all said it did not, we would be in a very odd position. We would have a hard time asserting confidently that ECT works. But there has been positive testimony from patients about ECT's efficacy throughout its history. I will show that much of this testimony even comes from patients with scathing complaints about, or even opposition to, the treatment.

There have been such patients with complaints throughout the history of ECT. Not only have there been persistent concerns about adverse effects, there are dark stories of abusive uses. No history of ECT can be complete without attending to both sides of this story. The historiography of therapeutics has grown since Rosenberg's lament, but where much of it has focused on efficacy, one of my goals here is to raise analogous questions about adverse effects. Just as efficacy is related to historical context, the meaning and significance of side effects are also historically variable.

While historians always like to be able to show that something thought of as ahistorical has a history, there is a larger significance to this argument. The very idea of a "side" effect, I will argue, is presupposed only by the recent rise of therapeutic specificity in biomedicine. That accomplishment led to dramatic clinical successes. It also led to a deep cultural change in how we think about medicine and what medicine is. We want our medicine to do no harm. But there are strong currents in American medical culture that push it to be aggressive as well.[34] We may have developed a cultural inability to acknowledge therapeutic procedures as double-edged.

Certainly, running electricity through the brain is not something healthy people should do. But healthy people also should not get the chemotherapy cancer patients get, or take the antiretroviral drugs AIDS patients use. Insulin is not prescribed to people who do not have diabetes. For that matter, it is not wise for a pain-free person to start taking a lot of Tylenol. ECT is used for severe mental illness, and even then not in a majority of cases. To consider ECT worth its risks—risks that are themselves hotly debated, although few doubt that any risks exist—means taking severe depression seriously as an illness. As we will see especially in Chapter Five, there have been those who have doubted the reality of all mental illness, and they have understandably been most critical of ECT. Some of them have, however, relied on an arbitrary definition of illness, a definition stressing visible lesions. This is, though, an arbitrary narrowing of the concept of illness beyond any typically found in medicine, modern lay culture, thousands of years of history, or cross-cultural comparison.

ECT and Medical Analogies

Is getting ECT just like going to the dentist? This may seem like a strange question, but the comparison is common. For example, ECT proponent Max Fink makes it in his accessible handbook of ECT for laypeople.[35] ECT patient Martha Manning, who wrote a memoir of her depressive illness and treatment by ECT, says her clinician made the comparison before she underwent the procedure. Manning writes of being shown a study

> in which a majority of ECT patients reported that it was no more distressing than 'a dental procedure.' Always the empiricist, I wonder what choices were offered to the participants. 'Was ECT more like having your eyes plucked out by vultures, or undergoing a simple dental procedure.'[36]

The comparison to the dentist suggests that getting ECT can be mildly unpleasant, but is really no big deal. This is not a very helpful way of talking about ECT, though. The vast majority of ECT patients are people in very acute suffering, taking what they perceive as a drastic step after other measures have failed. People rarely go to the dentist for severe or life-threatening conditions. And as unpleasant as a serious dental procedure can be, former dental patients generally do not say they feel they lost a part of their self afterward. There may be debate about the frequency of this complaint for ECT patients, but no one can deny that it sometimes occurs.

The puzzling nature of ECT—the mystery of how it works, its counter-intuitiveness to begin with—prompts analogies. When something is strange or difficult to understand, people will seek familiar points of comparison. As a controversial procedure, whose mechanism of efficacy is poorly understood, and whose risks are uncertain, ECT is enigmatic. This occasions analogies to other medical procedures we think we understand better. For critics of ECT practice, those analogies are barbaric relics of outdated medicine, such as leeching (which is still in use, and is more a symbolic marker of medical barbarism than a discredited practice). For ECT supporters, the analogies are with accepted, lauded medical advances; Shorter and Healy, for example, dub ECT the "penicillin of psychiatry."[37]

Both sets of analogies seek symbolic resonance in medicine's past, but they evoke only the superficial emotional tone of the treatment in question. Some medical historians now propose that leeching endured as a therapy because it could be safe and effective, so comparing it to ECT as a barbarism is misleading.[38] The opposite analogy, to penicillin, has the correspondingly opposite weakness. Penicillin's image is that of an unalloyed medical success, and that seems to be how Shorter and Healy intend the analogy. It is a misleading comparison, though, because penicillin is a cure, not simply a means of remitting symptoms. Furthermore, a more probing study of medical history shows that for all its virtues, penicillin has drawbacks, particularly when overused.[39] In this sense, the analogy may be a good one in ways that Shorter and Healy did not intend. Both the positive and negative analogies are less than helpfully revealing of ECT's place in the history and present of therapeutics.

The Patient's Perspective

In a statement advocating patient-centered histories of medicine, Roy Porter wrote:

> Medicine today is a supremely well-entrenched, prestigious profession, yoked to a body of relatively autonomous, self-directing science, expertise, and practices. It is hardly surprising, then, that it has tended to produce histories of itself cast in the mold of its own current image, stories of successive breakthroughs in medical science, heroic pioneers of

surgical techniques, of the supersession of ignorant folkloric remedies and barefaced charlatanry through the use of medicine as a liberal, ethical, corporate profession.[40]

Almost 20 years later, this observation seems dated, because the challenge to the heroic rendering has been successful within the field of medical history—although whether it has succeeded in changing the implicit historical understandings of clinicians or the lay public is more questionable. Within the field of the history of medicine, Porter's challenge has been so successful that historians wishing to depict medicine's history in terms of heroic breakthroughs, or the progress of science, may do so tentatively or apologetically.[41] And the value of capturing patients' perspectives is assumed.

We may need, however, more discussion of what capturing patients' perspectives means in practice. Porter implies that the history of patients will provide a needed challenge to stories of biomedical progress. Historians of patients have often been attracted to examples where their stories constituted challenges to medical authority.[42] This has been a benefit to medical historiography, but it is also incomplete. While not all historians of patient views have depicted them as dissident voices against the rise of biomedicine, it is fair to say that we do not have many histories of content or grateful patients. And whether regarded as the result of its clinical efficacy or its cultural hegemony, biomedicine is popular. The history of psychiatry has at once been one of the biggest contributors to patient-centered history and a field deeply influenced by one of the most influential critiques of medicine, the antipsychiatry movement.[43] Attempts to capture patients' voices in the history of medicine, and in the history of ECT, will surely be incomplete if it includes only those who raise voices of protest. But it will also be clear that a patients' history of ECT is not a simple tale of happy, satisfied customers. There is a commingling of gratitude and loss in patients' representations of their experience. This is what makes ECT's history complex, despite many renderings of it as simple.

ECT's Critics and Proponents

ECT has had many critics, and I want to stress at the outset that their views are not identical. There are those who regard mental illness as a myth and psychiatry itself as an imposition on human freedom and difference, who reject a medical model of what others call mental illness. This view may be most famously represented by Thomas Szasz, but he has been far from alone in articulating it. From this point of view, ECT might not only be seen as inappropriate but singled out as especially malign. Other critics of ECT include those who favor psychotherapy, but are opposed to virtually all somatic treatments. Narrowing the circle further would include those who do not object to the use of medications, but oppose ECT in all cases, and still further, those who think it should only be done when voluntary (although these may include some who think existing consent practices are inadequate).

Proponents of ECT have not been a unified block, either. There are a few who think it should be more of a front-line treatment than it is now, and others who accept the view, widely held now in psychiatry, that it should mainly be used only when medications and/or psychotherapy have failed. ECT proponents are unified, though, in believing ECT is effective in alleviating symptoms.

On Psychiatric Diagnosis

A specter haunts the history of psychiatry, the specter of diagnosis. One does not have to take the Szaszian view that mental illness is a myth to see that psychiatric diagnoses are in constant flux, their boundaries are porous, and they often reflect prevailing social orthodoxies rather than timeless and universal conceptions of sickness. So, when looking at a past diagnosis of "consumption" we may have relative ease (although not full certainty) in concluding the patient had what we now call "tuberculosis," but comparable translations are considered more fraught for psychiatry. Even when the same word is used, it is far from clear that we are seeing the same symptom cluster across eras. We do not know, for example, whether a patient with the diagnosis "schizophrenia" in the 1940s would get the same diagnosis with the same presentation today, and there are those who doubt it is a useful label altogether.

The account of ECT that follows is not invested in the validity of any nosology, past or present. When I use diagnostic language, I am only asserting that this was the diagnosis used, not accepting any judgments about its validity in general or its applicability to a particular case. I am simply making the empirical statement that the diagnostic label was applied. As I argued at length in my earlier work on colonial psychiatry, this caution does not preclude the acceptance of a medical model of psychic distress, any more than it requires it.[44] Still less does it require any doubt about the reality of the distress itself. There have been ECT patients who did not believe themselves to be ill. But many were clearly in acute pain whether they considered themselves ill or not.

What Is at Stake?

As debates over ECT have unfolded over the past 75 years or so, there have always been voices of moderation. Both patients and clinicians have cautioned against the dangers of exaggerating ECT's usefulness, harmlessness, or power to harm. But it will become clear that these voices have often been muffled in the polarization of the subject.

The story of this polarization in the United States commands attention for at least four reasons. First, it concerns human suffering. Reducing human suffering is one of the most inarguable goods, and if opinions differ as to whether ECT is important primarily because it alleviates or causes suffering, a complex historical account of precisely this problem seems called for. Second is the issue of informed consent. We now have a general consensus that if a medical procedure carries risks, patients need to be informed of those risks. But this is a challenge for ECT, partly because the highly fraught cultural associations with the treatment mean many potential patients bring misconceptions with them, but also because the degree of risk is not agreed upon even in the relevant scientific and clinical communities. A complex historical account of this problem also seems called for. Third, our ability to tolerate ambiguous stories seems to be limited. ECT has been depicted according to two of the most shopworn storylines in medical history: a technological breakthrough representing medical progress, and a practice of social control. Our grasp of the possibility that a single therapy can embody both of these storylines is impaired. Finally, I hope to show that human physiology is embedded in history. This is no longer a startling proposal among historians. A historiography of the human body began to take shape and grow in the 1980s—around the same time the revival of ECT was beginning, which may be more than coincidence.[45] But while this historiography has challenged the intuition that the body is a constant amidst cultural and political change, that intuition remains strong. The history of ECT can show that what might appear to be an immutable physical fact—what happens when you induce seizures in a human body?—is influenced by cultural context.

The tendency to treat the story of ECT as a simple one is a symptom of the way this therapy taps our greatest hopes for what medicine can be, as well as our deepest fears of what it might do to us. Going to the doctor, placing oneself and one's body in the hands of an expert, is an act of trust. We do it because we suffer, and we know and hope medicine can allay suffering. But we also know and fear that medicine can be used to control us, and experiment on us.

By turning my attention to the controversies over ECT, I am not claiming this provides me with an objectivity so far not achieved. Nor do I claim to be neutral about the arguments. One does not study something for a long time without forming opinions about it. Rather, I hope to show that examining the controversy over ECT allows a greater yield of understanding of these larger questions about medicine, particularly American medicine. The international nature of psychiatry requires me to make some forays into figures and events in other countries, but I have selected them according to the criterion of whether they were important for American debates.

The format of this book is deliberately more thematic than chronological. Put abstractly, it hinges on four major themes: time, power, person, and evidence. With regard to time, I want to show first of all that while the linear and heroic conception of progress in medical history has been rightly dislodged, there may be costs and limitations in replacing it with its simple negation. Also regarding time: in psychiatric history especially, a dominant metaphor for understanding historical time has been one of a pendulum, as we imagine the history swinging back and forth between emphasis on mind and emphasis on body. As I show especially in Chapter Four, this way of thinking about the history of psychiatry can obscure as much as it reveals.

As to power, the controversies over ECT have often revolved around two questions. In its early decades, its power to heal was pitted in public debate against its power to control—that is, to enforce social disciplines of various kinds. And there have also been continual debates pitting ECT's power to heal against its power to harm, although as we will see the emphasis of these debates has changed over time. What I will show, though, is that in both cases—healing versus controlling, healing versus harming—the opposing pairs have often combined in intricate ways that have too rarely been acknowledged by partisans. This matters in a field of debate so often framed in the fiercest of either/ors.

Debates over what kind of psychiatry we ought to have—one dominated by talk therapies or one by somatic treatments—are also debates over what we are, fundamentally as people. The tension between these two ways of thinking of the person has pulled at all of psychiatric history. But it has had a special importance for ECT because of the undoubted intensity of ECTs effects, although these effects are alarming to some and emboldening to others.

Finally, regarding evidence, this book will be juxtaposing evidence from science, including quantitative studies, with more subjective and narrative evidence. My approach is not to treat them the same, but to treat them both with respect. Science is imperfect, springs from social sources, and does not attain perfect objectivity. This does not mean we cannot recognize good method, or that we can glibly reject scientific findings as social constructions. On the other hand, there are, I will argue, aspects of patient experience that may not be well captured in scientific and quantitative studies.

ECT is a fairly simple technology that has survived into an era of very sophisticated medical science. Its development was based on a clinical premise now considered to be false. Its early use was based on limited observations of very small numbers of patients, and it has survived into the era of large-scale, double-blind, randomized clinical trials. It was invented at a time when the medicinal uses of mood-altering agents was rare, and has continued into a time when they are ubiquitous. Yet ECT is a very powerful technology. Understanding why this power continues to be idealized or vilified demands an account that tolerates ambiguity and uncertainty.

Notes

1 Karen V. Kukil, ed., *The Unabridged Journals of Sylvia Plath, 1950–1962* (New York: Anchor Books, 2000), 455.
2 Sylvia Plath, *The Bell Jar* (New York: Bantam Books, 1971), 117–118.
3 Roy Porter, *The Faber Book of Madness* (London: Faber and Faber, 1991), 336.

4 Kukil, ed., *The Unabridged Journals of Sylvia Plath,* 455. See also Alex Beam, *Gracefully Insane: The Rise and Fall of America's Premier Mental Hospital* (New York: PublicAffairs, 2001), 152.

5 Beam, *Gracefully Insane,* 154. See also Anne Stevenson, *Bitter Fame: A Life of Sylvia Plath* (Boston: Houghton Mifflin, 1989), 43–49.

6 I believe ch. 5 of Joel Braslow's *Mental Ills and Bodily Cures: Psychiatric Treatment in the First Half of the Twentieth Century* (Berkeley: University of California, 1997) remains the best historical account of ECT. Although deliberately focused in time and space, it acknowledges the ambiguities of ECT's history more than subsequent scholarship. Since its publication, there have been two book-length scholarly treatments: Timothy W. Kneeland and Carol A. B. Warren, *Pushbutton Psychiatry: A History of Electroshock in America* (Westport: Praeger Publishers, 2002) and Edward Shorter and David Healy, *Shock Therapy: A History of Electroconvulsive Treatment in Mental Illness* (New Brunswick: Rutgers University Press, 2007). See also Kitty Dukakis and Larry Tye, *Shock: The Healing Power of Electroconvulsive Therapy* (New York: Penguin, 2006) and Linda Andre, *Doctors of Deception: What They Don't Want You to Know about Shock Therapy* (New Brunswick: Rutgers University Press, 2009).

7 Max Fink and Charles Kellner, "The Perplexing History of ECT in Three Books," *Psychiatric Times,* August 12, 2010.

8 Many ECT proponents and practitioners do acknowledge that the treatment is controversial. See, for example, Julian Bustin, Mark J. Rapoport, Murali Krishna, Daniel Matusevich, Carlos Finkelsztein, Sergio Strejilevich, and David Anderson, "Are Patients' Attitudes towards and Knowledge of Electroconvulsive Therapy Transcultural? A Multi-National Pilot Study," *International Journal of Geriatric Psychiatry* 23 (2008) 497–503.

9 This usage and the practices associated with it are the subject of searching critique in Naomi Klein, *The Shock Doctrine: The Rise of Disaster Capitalism* (New York: Henry Holt and Company, 2007).

10 In the early decades, clinicians also used the similar term "electrical stimulation therapy" or "EST," but this term was mostly abandoned by the 1960s.

11 Kneeland and Warren, *Pushbutton Psychiatry;* Shorter and Healy, *Shock Therapy.*

12 Margaret Rowbottom and Charles Susskind, *Electricity and Medicine: History of Their Interaction* (San Francisco: San Francisco Press, 1984).

13 See the epigram by eighteenth-century author William Battie, reproduced at the beginning of Max Fink, "Induced Seizures and Human Behavior," in Fink, ed., *Psychobiology of Convulsive Therapy* (New York: V. H. Winston & Sons, 1974), 1.

14 See Shorter, *A History of Psychiatry,* 214–217, for one account.

15 In the first major textbook on shock treatments, Kalinowsky and Hoch said that the chemical shock therapies should still be learned by psychiatrists, and sometimes used, although they did not explain why, given the advantages of ECT that they stressed. Lothar B. Kalinowsky and Paul H. Hoch, *Shock Treatments and Other Somatic Procedures in Psychiatry* (New York: Grune and Stratton, 1946), 103.

16 Kalinowsky and Hoch, *Shock Treatments,* 103.

17 Joel Braslow, *Mental Ills and Bodily Cures: Psychiatric Treatment in the First Half of the Twentieth Century* (Berkeley: University of California, 1997), 99–123; G. E. Burns, "The Scientific Origins of Electroconvulsive Therapy: A Conceptual History," *History of Psychiatry* viii (1997) 105–119; Norman S. Endler, "The Origins of Electroconvulsive Therapy (ECT)," *Convulsive Therapy* 4, 1 (1988) 5–23; Luca Alverno, "The Origins of Electroconvulsive Therapy," *Wisconsin Medical Journal* (February 1990) 54–56.

18 There are some exceptions to this. For example, ECT is often recommended as a first-line treatment for pregnant women with severe mood disorders. ECT is also considered very effective in the treatment of catatonia.

19 Charles E. Rosenberg, "The Therapeutic Revolution: Medicine, Meaning, and Social Change in Nineteenth-Century America," in Morris J. Vogel and Charles E. Rosenberg, eds., *The Therapeutic Revolution: Essays in the Social History of American Medicine* (Philadelphia: University of Pennsylvania Press, 1979), 3–23.

20 The anthropological literature on therapeutic efficacy is large, probably larger than the historical literature. For a précis and taxonomy of the anthropology, see Thomas Csordas, *The Sacred Self: A Cultural Phenomenology of Charismatic Healing* (Berkeley: University of California Press, 1994), 2–3. Csordas identifies four distinct theories of ritual healing, all of which proceed from the assumption that ritual healing does, in fact, heal.

21 John Harley Warner, *The Therapeutic Perspective: Medical Practice, Knowledge, and Identity in America, 1820–1885* (Princeton: Princeton University Press, 1997, originally published 1986). In the preface to the second edition, Warner responds to a review by Steven Shapin that lamented Warner's unwillingness to draw the most relativist conclusions from his material.

22 Jack D. Pressman, *Last Resort: Psychosurgery and the Limits of Medicine* (Cambridge: Cambridge University Press, 1998), 5.

23 See Pressman, *Last Resort,* 10. Terming the procedure "drastic" itself introduces the kind of presentism Pressman is trying to write against, as treatments considered drastic in one era might not be in another. Pressman's discussion of Rosenberg also omits mention of the endorsement of medical progress that concludes Rosenberg's essay.

24 Braslow, *Mental Ills,* 4.

25 One rich field for study along these lines has been the medicalization of childbirth. See Emily Martin, *The Woman in the Body: A Cultural Analysis of Reproduction* (Boston: Beacon Press, 1987) and Robbie E. Davis-Floyd, *Birth as an American Rite of Passage* (2nd edition, Berkeley: University of California Press, 2003).

26 An exception is Jeremy Greene's *Prescribing by Numbers: Drugs and the Definition of Disease* (Baltimore: The Johns Hopkins University Press, 2007), an insightful study of the use of drugs to not only treat, but to re-define, chronic illnesses.

27 Shorter and Healy, *Shock Therapy,* 214.

28 On the historical development of clinical trials, see Harry Marks, *The Progress of Experiment: Science and Therapeutic Reform in the United States, 1900–1990* (Cambridge: Cambridge University Press, 1997).

29 For a review essay summarizing many of the findings on efficacy, see Robert M. Greenberg and Charles H. Kellner, "Electroconvulsive Therapy: A Selected Review," *American Journal of Geriatric Psychiatry* 13, 4 (April 2005) 268–281.

30 Greenberg and Kellner, "Electroconvulsive Therapy: A Selected Review," 268.

31 Greenberg and Kellner, "Electroconvulsive Therapy: A Selected Review," 268.

32 Greenberg and Kellner, "Electroconvulsive Therapy: A Selected Review," 269.

33 This point is made with regard to ECT in Steve Baldwin and Melissa Oxlad, *Electroshock and Minors: A Fifty-Year Review* (Westport: Greenwood Press, 2000), 103.

34 See Lynn Payer, *Medicine and Culture* (New York: Penguin Books, 1988).

35 Max Fink, *Electroshock: Restoring the Mind* (New York: Oxford University Press, 1999), 4.

36 Martha Manning, *Undercurrents: A Life beneath the Surface* (New York: HarperSanFrancisco, 1994), 102.

37 Shorter and Healy, *Shock Therapy,* 144.
38 On leeching, see for example Noga Arikha, *Passions and Tempers: A History of the Humours* (New York: Harper Perennial, 2007), 90–91.
39 See Robert Bud, *Penicillin: Triumph and Tragedy* (Oxford: Oxford University Press, 2007).
40 Roy Porter, "The Patient's View: Doing Medical History from Below," *Theory and Society* 14, 2 (March 1985) 175–198. The quote appears on page 175. For a critique and contextualization of Porter's article from a somewhat different angle from mine, see the editors' introduction to L. Stephen Jacyna and Stephen T. Casper, *The Neurological Patient in History* (Rochester: University of Rochester Press, 2012), 3.
41 In advice for medical students planning to do historical research, Jacalyn Duffin (only half-jokingly, I think) suggests that if they are tempted to use the word "progress," they should "take a deep breath, and if that doesn't work, take a Valium." Jacalyn Duffin, *History of Medicine: A Scandalously Short Introduction* (Toronto: University of Toronto Press, 1999), 374.
42 For an example in the history of psychiatry, see Geoffrey Reaume, *Remembrance of Patients Past: Patient Life at the Toronto Hospital for the Insane, 1870–1940* (Oxford: Oxford University Press, 2000).
43 The antipsychiatry movement is one that has influenced historians more than historians have analyzed or historicized it, although there are a few exceptions. A very good recent contribution is Michael E. Staub, *Madness Is Civilization: When the Diagnosis Was Social, 1948–1980* (Chicago: University of Chicago Press, 2011).
      The final chapter of Elaine Showalter's *The Female Malady* (New York: Viking, 1985) is a compelling feminist critique of antipsychiatry as practiced by R.D. Laing. Norman Dain has examined antipsychiatry in "Psychiatry and Anti-Psychiatry in the United States" in Mark S. Micale and Roy Porter, eds., *Discovering the History of Psychiatry* (Oxford: Oxford University Press, 1994) and "Antipsychiatry," in Roy W. Menninger and John C. Nemaha, eds., *American Psychiatry After World War II, 1944–1994.* David Healy's *The Creation of Psychopharmacology* (Cambridge: Harvard University Press, 1992) is notable for showing some of the impact antipsychiatry has had on mainstream biopsychiatry.
44 Jonathan Sadowsky, *Imperial Bedlam: Institutions of Madness and Colonialism in Southwest Nigeria* (Berkeley: University of California Press, 1999).
45 The literature on the history of the body is by now very large, but for one important example from when it was relatively new see Thomas Laqueur, *Making Sex: Body and Gender from the Greeks to Freud* (Cambridge: Harvard University Press, 1990).

1 Origins and Origin Myths

As knowledge of electricity grew in modern Western societies, an ambivalent fascination developed. A mysterious force with unknown and seemingly limitless potential, some thought it the source or essence of life itself. By that measure, it was also something to be feared. Witness the birth of such a monster:

> It was on a dreary night of November that I beheld the accomplishment of my toils. With an anxiety that almost amounted to agony, I collected the instruments of life around me, that I might infuse a spark of being into the lifeless thing that lay at my feet . . . I saw the dull yellow eye of the creature open; it breathed hard, and a convulsive motion agitated its limbs.[1]

A spark, a convulsion, a lifeless form brought to life: although the doctor here, in Mary Shelley's *Frankenstein,* is trying to bring to life matter that is literally dead, rather than suffering the figurative death of severe mental illness, the passage is eerily similar to ECT in certain respects.

In the novel, upon encountering Doctor Frankenstein later, the monster describes the period following his awakening in terms that could well have come from an ECT patient, without even a change in diction:

> It is with considerable difficulty that I remember the original era of my being; the events of that period appear confused and indistinct. A strange multiplicity of sensations seized me, and I saw, felt, heard, and smelt at the same time . . .[2]

The reason to raise the Frankenstein story in connection with ECT is not, however, to suggest that Shelley somehow anticipated the therapy or influenced its development. It does, however, show that before ECT was invented, its main ingredient—electricity—had rich connotations with modernity, Romanticism, and also with mad science, science gone haywire—although, as Susan Lederer has argued, the monster's sensitivity and other details from the story suggest that Shelley had a more nuanced agenda.[3] And cultural associations between this scene and ECT may run very deep. In the film version of *One Flew Over the Cuckoo's Nest,* the protagonist returns to the ward from his ECT treatment, walking with what had become cinematically familiar as the Frankenstein monster gait.[4] But this association does not show that resistance to ECT can be reduced to an irrational cultural memory. Not only would this misread the history of ECT, it would misread the significance of the Frankenstein story. Scientific and medical progress is double-edged, and this is why Shelley's story has resonance.

Electricity and the Body

Electroconvulsive therapy is a dense term, and even the question of which part of it should be stressed is potentially controversial. From a historical point of view, is it ELECTRO-convulsive therapy, one best placed in the history of uses of electricity in medicine?[5] Or is it electro-CONVULSIVE therapy, one best placed in the history of induced convulsions?[6] Electrical treatments for mental illnesses have a long history, dating back at least to the eighteenth century, and they have had a variety of clinical rationales. These various rationales have included aversive therapy (creating unpleasant associations with an impulse or activity), replenishing life force, and simple fright. Inducing convulsions, though, had a completely different rationale. Meduna's chemical convulsive therapy was based on the proposed antagonism between schizophrenia and epilepsy. This is one of those areas, though, where polarized debate conceals the complexity. ECT's clinical origins cannot be cordoned off from the history of electricity in medicine, and regarded simply as a technical modification of other convulsive therapies. But even if it could, the history of electricity and its relationship to the human body would remain relevant, because it is a source and reflection of ambivalent cultural symbolism about what our bodies and minds are made from, and who we are. Placing ECT's origins solely in the tradition of electrical therapies, however, would require us to ignore the clinical rationale—what early practitioners thought they were doing, and why—entirely.

From the beginnings of European progress in harnessing electricity for practical technologies, it was applied to human bodies. And in these beginnings, it was seen as both a source of danger and a source—perhaps *the* source—of life itself.[7] In the early nineteenth century, there were experiments to test whether electricity could be used even to resurrect dead human bodies, and it was in the context of experiments like this that Shelley could imagine the Frankenstein story.

Electricity between Spirit and Matter

When the American colonies were being settled, European science was growing interest in electricity.[8] As Europe and the United States industrialized, electricity became, *par excellence,* a symbol of scientific advance and wonder.[9] It also became deeply associated with life, and in some representations, the secret of life itself. Not surprisingly, this led to attempts to use it medicinally, and for many conditions, medical treatments were to be touted as miracle cures. Indeed—and I love this detail—in 1744 a German professor concluded that because electricity must be useful, and there is no use for it in theology or law, it must therefore be useful for medicine.[10] There was no more fertile area for these hopes than nervous conditions, as the nervous system came to be seen as pre-eminently electrical, often analogized to the emerging telegraph system.[11] Yet amid these positive associations, electrotherapeutics were shot through with controversy from their beginning and throughout their history. Hyperbolic therapeutic claims of early enthusiasts prompted skeptical counter-claims. Early eighteenth-century medical uses aroused suspicion at both London's Royal Society and Paris's Academy of Sciences. There were counter-currents accompanying any associations of electricity with a positive vision of modernity, and cultural associations of electricity soon became linked with fringe or quack science, and at worst with terror, and death.

Medicinal uses of electricity continued. These included attempts to cure cases of paralysis, for example.[12] But the skepticism of much of the scientific establishment was continuous. Electricity was so frequently presented as a panacea that those who wished to make it more respectable had constantly to distance themselves from zealots, and to insist that its uses were limited.[13] Each new generation of electrical practitioners claimed to be the one that would establish the reputability of electrical cures.[14] This was partly the intent of pioneer electrical scientist Luigi Galvani, who showed in the late eighteenth century that he could produce electricity from animal tissue; a frog's legs twitched convulsively when nerve and muscle were connected through a metallic circuit.[15] Galvani did not introduce any new techniques to electrical medicine, but he believed he had established its physiological basis, and his work did help to further its respectability.[16]

Galvani's finding also encouraged developing ideas that electricity was in some way the secret of life, what differentiated animate matter from inanimate. What this meant was debatable, though. For some, the link between life and electricity provided support for the most materialist conceptions of human life and the denial of the existence of the soul.[17] This was connected to an emergent view of the human body as a machine.[18] For conservatives such as Edmund Burke, this was precisely the problem with linking electricity and the body. Burke's concerns were justified, because many nineteenth-century radicals were indeed inspired by the link between electricity and the body, and the malleability of humanity that might imply. British electrical scientist Michael Faraday sought to debunk the idea that electricity was the basic stuff of life, arguing that if it were, it would not be possible to experiment with it.[19] For Faraday, this argument was critical to promoting the respectability of electrical science, creating distance between the science and its potential radical taint. Samuel Taylor Coleridge and some of his medical contemporaries articulated a middle position, seeing electricity as a mediator between the body and the soul.[20] Morus points out that while European observers might agree that electricity was a powerful force, "by the second decade of the nineteenth century, galvanism had already acquired a dangerous history and a dodgy reputation. It was at once the plaything of fashionable dilettantes, the hope of radical firebrands, and the *bête noire* of conservative ideologies anxious to stamp out anything that seemed to smack of atheism, materialism and all such French connections."[21] Morus also shows that electricity was used in nineteenth-century Britain to induce convulsions in dead bodies, to see if the corpses could be revived. This—along with the practice of snatching corpses for investigative dissections—forms the background to Shelley's fantasy novel. For example, Morus tells the story of the body of Tom Weems, whose corpse was electrified in an effort to disprove the theory that human bodies could be re-animated electrically.

American electrical science followed European in seeking practical medical applications.[22] Electrical shocks were used in the eighteenth century to resuscitate in cases of cardiac arrest.[23] The great and iconic early American scientist of electricity was, of course, Benjamin Franklin. Franklin also experimented with medical applications of electricity to the body. Franklin and some of his contemporaries believed that electrical shocks—to induce convulsions—could be used to treat melancholia, the term used for depression before the twentieth century. Franklin's highly pragmatic and anti-metaphysical approach was not the only one in North America, though. For Dr. T. Gale, who wrote the first major statement on medical electricity in North America, electricity was the mediator between the divine and material worlds.[24] Gale treated hundreds of cases, claiming success with cases of hysteria, epilepsy, fevers, and inflammation, believing he was rejuvenating the nervous system with this divine gift. And, in the late eighteenth century, a woman claiming to be possessed by a demon sought help from Joseph Priestly himself, who cured her with an electrical machine.

In the United States, the decades before the invention of ECT was the time when electricity stopped being an exotic and mysterious aspect of nature, detached from daily life for most people. Instead, it colonized daily life, transforming everything: homes, factories, businesses, and toys.[25] Between 1850 and 1950, the United States became the leading energy consumer in the world.[26] But electricity did not cease being an object of wonder as it became part of everyday life. As David Nye has shown, electricity was not simply a utility or a technology, but a culturally fraught symbol of modern life—and in particular, of progress. Electricity was, Nye says, "the wonder of the age, the hallmark of progress," "a mysterious power Americans had long connected to magnetism, the nervous system, heat, power, lightning, sex, health, and light."[27] As electrification spread, it was a linchpin of optimistic thinking of the future, as people imagined the work it might save and the conveniences it might bring.

But there were also more somber sides to electrification. It was useful for social control: lighting and alarms could deter trespassers, bells on clocks could be used to increase time discipline for workers, and most gruesomely, electrification provided a new mode of execution. Nye points out that anti-modernists would highlight some of these developments, and focus on electricity's powers for "subjection and destruction."[28] But he also emphasizes that this was a counter-current; dominant cultural associations were positive. Most people saw the spread of electricity as a triumph of science over superstition.[29] New good ideas came to be represented by a light bulb over the head.

While electricity came to be seen as a source of life, perhaps even in some way life itself, this led to new conceptions of body and self. American English became peppered with new idioms, Nye shows: an energetic person was a "human dynamo," a performance was "electrifying," and an angry person could "blow a fuse." People were beings that could be "plugged in" or "juiced up" and even turned on and off. The psychological implications were profound. The human personality was now an electrical system that could be "switched on," "overloaded," and "burned out."[30]

As electrical power became more widely available, a range of medical practitioners touted it as a cure for virtually anything. Both in office care and home use, electrical belts and other devices were a brisk business.[31] The conditions treated in some way with electricity over the course of the nineteenth and early twentieth centuries included infectious diseases such as cholera and tuberculosis, epilepsy, strokes, deafness, blindness, gout, female hirsuteness, and sexual impotence, to name just a few of many examples.[32] Doubts modern readers might have about the efficacy of some of these treatments were voiced by contemporary critics. Many who considered themselves regular medical practitioners denounced the spread of electrical cures as quackery. But as medical historians have pointed out, the border between regular medicine and fringe medicine and quackery has always been a porous one, and was far more porous in this era than it is now.[33] De la Pena observes that many patients reported great results from electrical devices in situations we might now consider unlikely, which she attributes to placebo effects. In an era before the routine scrutiny of randomized clinical trials, the evidence of experience counted for much.

Electrical conceptions of body and self were embedded in the signature mental illness of late Victorian America, neurasthenia. This era was also marked by its attention to hysteria, but hysteria was more closely associated with sites in continental Europe, such as Paris and Vienna, and hysteria was also an ancient malady.[34] Neurasthenia was the paradigmatic mental affliction of burgeoning American modernity. The illness became a sensational national preoccupation. Alienist George Beard did not invent the term, but as Shorter puts it, "he launched it on its century-long worldwide trajectory."[35] The term literally meant "tired nerves," and was considered to be a depletion of nerve force due to the stresses of modern living.[36] Over the course of its career, neurasthenia became something of a wastebasket category, with varying symptomatology. His treatment for and writing on the subject made Beard one of the most famous physicians of his era.

For Beard, electricity was both the source and the cure for neurasthenia. His 1880 book *American Nervousness* blamed Edison for the overstimulation of modern life. But Beard's treatment program—contrasting strongly with the "rest cure" advocated by his prominent contemporary Silas Weir Mitchell—centered on the belief that applying electricity to the body would act as the necessary restorative.[37]

So electricity had a rich medical and psychiatric history in the United States well before ECT. But this hardly prepared the cultural ground for an easy introduction of ECT. Although Beard's use did help to provide electrotherapy with some respectability, electrotherapy would retain some association with quackery. And of course, the fact remains that applying electricity to a human body can be dangerous or lethal, and became deliberately so in the late nineteenth century with the introduction of the electric chair—since used almost exclusively in the United States—as a method of execution.[38] Disturbing associations with electricity did not come only from realms outside of psychiatry. In World War I, intentionally brutal and coercive psychiatric uses of electricity were made in an effort to make psychiatric illness at least as unpleasant as war itself.

ECT and the History of Somatic Psychiatry[39]

If you have read Allen Ginsberg's poem "Howl" without knowing the history of psychiatry, some passages may be puzzling. Ginsberg makes references to hydrotherapy, occupational therapy, insulin, electricity, Metrazol, and other forms of therapy, and in the staccato, elliptical style of the poem, associates them with amnesia.[40] These lines are actually a compressed, and bitter, history of institutional psychiatric treatments in the first half of the twentieth century.

When convulsive therapy for mental illness was invented in the 1930s, biomedicine was in a period of growing self-confidence. One vivid emblem of medicine's success was the introduction of penicillin, which capped a half-century of remarkable scientific advance in understanding, preventing, and treating infectious disease. This advance spurred, in industrial countries, what may have been the greatest reduction in mortality in human history.[41] Medicine's prestige was high, as knowledge of the achievements flowing from germ theory permeated the worldview of laypeople.[42] Psychiatry's prestige and cultural impact was also increasing. People increasingly turned to psychiatry for solutions to problems in living.[43] But psychiatry never quite radiated the same aura of progress. The reason for this is simple. It was not having comparable clinical success. Sanitation, nutrition, and therapeutic advance all reduced morbidity and mortality from infectious disease. Psychiatry was providing temporary palliatives, at best. People with severe mental illnesses were housed in asylums and hospitals, which were ever more overcrowded.

Despite its comparative therapeutic ineffectiveness, the half-century before ECT was a time of rising optimism in psychiatry. This optimism was reflected in three developments. First was the rise of "dynamic" psychiatry and related psychotherapies, represented most vigorously by Freudian psychoanalysis. Throughout the history of these treatments, there have been skeptics of their efficacy. This skepticism has been amplified since the rise of second-wave biological psychiatry in the late twentieth century. And as Freud himself conceded, there was little that insight-oriented therapy could do for severe mental illnesses such as psychoses. Even with these doubts and limitations, in the first half of the twentieth century belief in the efficacy of psychoanalysis was widespread, both within medicine and among the lay public, leading to W. H. Auden's characterization of Freudianism as "a whole climate of opinion."[44] This belief helped lay the groundwork for the second development reflecting psychiatric optimism, the mental hygiene movement. This movement attempted to expand psychiatry's scope, so that it would no longer be a service for the severely ill or disabled, but rather a broad endeavor, both preventive and curative, to increase the mental health of the wider population. The third development of psychiatric optimism was the rise of the new somatic treatments.

The success of vaccines, and later antibiotics, led psychiatrists to seek similar interventions on the bodies of sick people. The discovery of the linkage between syphilis and paresis offered the hope that all mental illnesses might have straightforward organic etiologies and cures. This was not so much a new idea as a new hopefulness. The use of relatively direct interventions on the body to treat madness is both long-standing and cross-culturally common. They were, for example, addressed in the Hippocratic corpus. So the attempts by critics of psychiatry such as Thomas Szasz to sever psychiatry from medicine run against not only recent psychiatric entrepreneurship, but also long and widely held precedents.[45] And, as madness has been widely recognized as a medical problem, it has always been treated both with seemingly physical means such as drugs and other bodily interventions, as well as spiritual, moral, behavioral, ritualistic—all the means we might now classify as "talk."

The first decades of the twentieth century were a time of restless innovation in psychiatry, yielding not only the growth of psychoanalysis and psychotherapy, but also a number of somatic treatments that are now mostly discarded.[46] The rise of psychopharmacology since the 1980s has, unsurprisingly, been accompanied by a growth in the historiography of somatic treatments.[47] One achievement of this new historiography has been to rescue discarded somatic treatments such as lobotomy, insulin coma therapy, and chemical convulsive therapies from what E. P. Thompson famously called "the enormous condescension of posterity."[48] Treatments that had sometimes been viewed as curiosities, forms of social control, or outright barbarism have been re-evaluated, with a new appreciation of their scientific rationale and even clinical utility. At its best, this historiography has achieved that most sacred of historians' goals: the reconstruction of proper context. The recent historiography has usually been more critical of surviving somatic treatments, such as the antidepressant and antipsychotic medications. Sympathetic restoration of context has been more generously applied to the treatments medicine has cast off.[49]

Many of the somatic treatments developed between the 1920s and 1950s were no doubt dangerous. And they were often tested on a captive asylum population in conditions lacking the informed consent standards we hope for today.[50] Some psychoanalysts went so far as to speculate that these somatic treatments reflected unconscious sadism toward the mentally ill, although there were also psychoanalysts who found them to be helpful adjuncts. But the experimenters were usually adhering to the same empirical and ethical standards that helped advance biomedicine—testing hypotheses, in order to try to find remedies for serious and often chronic distress. And while some treatments might seem in retrospect like extreme measures, their adoption cannot be seen as representing only the imperial ambitions of doctors. Chronic mental illness is devastating for patients and their families. In circumstances marked by desperation, people could be supportive of physicians' efforts to do something, anything.[51]

The twentieth-century treatments come in a succession that has become canonical in overviews, many of them associated with a particular innovator. The major developments include hydrotherapy; the prolonged sleep therapy developed by Jakob Klaesi in Zurich from 1920; Julius Wagner-Jauregg's malaria fever therapy for neurosyphilis, developed in Vienna in the 1920s; insulin coma therapy, pioneered by Manfred Sakel in Berlin in 1930; chemical convulsive therapy, championed by Ladislas von Meduna in Budapest in 1934; lobotomy, developed by Egas Moniz in Lisbon in 1935; and electroconvulsive therapy, invented by Ugo Cerletti and Lucio Bini in Rome in 1938. All of these treatments were announced as clinical successes, although for the most part they were not subject to clinical trials, which would become the gold standard for efficacy research after World War II. This canon usually omits one of the most important developments, namely the use of amphetamine to treat depression. This was particularly promoted by Boston psychiatrist Abraham Myerson in the 1930s. As Nicolas Rasmussen has shown, amphetamine has a claim to be the first psychopharmaceutical. He also shows that clinical trials were used to establish its efficacy.[52]

The history of somatic treatments is replete with new therapies hailed as a departure from previous practices deemed inhumane or coercive, only to be regarded themselves as inhumane and coercive in retrospect. Hydrotherapy is an example. It refers to an array of uses for water that were widely used in the late nineteenth and early twentieth centuries, including the continuous bath and the wet sheet pack. For the wet sheet pack, patients were wrapped tightly in sheets, at gradually rising temperatures. For continuous baths, patients were fastened to a hammock and placed in a tub, which was then covered in canvas, leaving just a hole for the head.[53] These highly restraining procedures were actually praised for being departures from the use of restraints. As Braslow's account makes clear, physicians favored the hydrotherapies precisely because they allowed doctors to control the behavior of the patients. And patients resisted them, sometimes strenuously.

The subtle point here is that the line between control and therapy is not neat. Sometimes therapies may appear to be more for the convenience of the doctors, or the patients' families, or the wider society, than for easing the suffering of the afflicted. And we can identify different levels of coerciveness not only among treatments, but in their application. To some extent, treating madness is inherently a way of controlling people who felt, or were felt by others, to be out of control. People who are suffering from morbid paranoid delusions that are disrupting family relations, or from catatonic depression that prevents any effective work or creative activity, may receive a treatment that increases their subjective sense of well-being, and allows them to improve familial relations and prosper in a fulfilling career. No doubt this can in some way accurately be called "social control," but there not always much moral or analytic gain in doing so. There are always important questions to ask about the physical, psychic, or financial costs of the treatment. There are also undoubtedly instances where psychiatric interventions are used in troubling ways to silence dissent, sometimes intentionally, and sometimes not. And finally, there is no question that many treatments can be used in punishing and coercive ways. But these are issues that need to be weighed in specific instances. A psychiatric treatment is not coercive in a sinister way simply because it returns a person to their expected social role, any more than it is coercive simply because it is somatic.

Wagner-Jauregg, who had been among those administering shocks to soldiers during World War I, had also been exploring the use of infectious agents that cause fevers for the use of psychiatric conditions since the 1880s. In 1917, he first treated a patient with neurosyphilis, and shortly thereafter reported success with nine patients.[54] Although a scary, painful, and risky treatment, malaria fever therapy was considered efficacious, not just by physicians, but by patients.[55] Malaria fever therapy was the first treatment in psychiatry to garner the Nobel Prize for Medicine. It has become axiomatic in the history of psychiatry to note how important malaria fever therapy was for establishing the optimistic precedent that somatic interventions could actually work. But it also established another optimistic precedent, as the treatment was used for an extremely wide variety of mental illnesses.[56] This pattern would repeat with electroconvulsive therapy, which in its early years was tried for a wide range of categories that were called mental illnesses, until its use was narrowed, mostly, to the management of affective disorders—an indication for which it had not been originally developed. Lobotomy would also be used for a wide range of diagnoses.[57]

The shock therapies are conventionally grouped as insulin coma therapy, chemical convulsive therapy, and electroconvulsive therapy. Historians have not imposed this grouping; the psychiatric profession used it when these therapies were developed.[58] How exactly they constitute a group is less obvious than one might think, but they were all motivated by a belief that severe mental illness required a major shock to the physical and psychical entity, to break through the illness to the person.

Insulin coma therapy was the first, developed by Manfred Sakel in Berlin. Sakel was experimenting with the use of insulin to treat addicts, and sometimes inadvertently induced hypoglycemic coma. Sakel found that for many of these patients, desire for alcohol disappeared, as did symptoms of agitation. He theorized that insulin coma might cure schizophrenia. When he tried it, he reported a success rate of 70%. Mental hospitals throughout the industrialized world adopted insulin coma therapy.[59] Its foundations were shaky, though. Doctors who used it often reported symptom remission, but if it was effective, its mechanism was unknown. Some of the patients experienced convulsions, and while Sakel himself believed the convulsions were the effective part of the treatment, there was no consensus about this among clinicians. What was clear was that the procedure was dangerous. Patients died at a rate of 2–5%.[60]

Insulin coma therapy was largely forgotten by the lay public. It did not, over the second half of the twentieth century, become a feature of popular imagination of psychiatry in the way that lobotomy and ECT did. It did figure in Sylvia Nasar's 1998 bestseller about mathematician John Nash, *A Beautiful Mind,* and its film adaptation.[61] Nash described the insulin treatment he received in a public hospital as "torture," but would also say later that he benefited from it, explicitly contrasting it with an ineffective Freudian treatment he had earlier received at McClean Hospital.[62] Nash's wife, Alicia, was determined to preserve his genius and sought for as long as possible to avoid drug or shock treatments, and particularly worried that ECT would damage his memory.[63]

The reason for the efficacy of insulin coma therapy may have been debated, but Ladislas von Meduna, the Hungarian physician who developed Metrazol therapy, was looking specifically for a way to induce convulsions. He and some contemporaries believed that epilepsy and schizophrenia were inversely correlated, a now-discredited premise. Meduna reasoned that if the symptoms of epilepsy could be induced in psychotic patients, their psychosis would remit. He first used camphor oil, before adopting a chemical known as Metrazol. The psychiatric profession was generally enthusiastic about Metrazol, and it too was widely adopted in hospitals. But while there were many reports of patients whose symptoms remitted, patients hated Metrazol therapy, almost universally. Doctors and nurses had to go to great lengths to get patients to swallow the medicine. In particular, patients often reported feelings of terror during the short interlude between swallowing the medicine and the beginning of the convulsions. This was why Cerletti looked for another way to induce the convulsions.

Lobotomy was developed around the same time as convulsive therapy, and has always been linked with it in public imagination. Lobotomy was first developed in Portugal by Egas Moniz, who then received the second, and so far the last, Nobel Prize in Medicine for a psychiatric intervention. Walter Freeman promoted it zealously in the United States. There were variations of the procedure, but all its forms consisted mainly of cutting connections between the pre-frontal cortex and other parts of the brain. Psychiatrists were enormously impressed by the power of lobotomy to provide a sense of calm relief to highly agitated patients. A simple, one-time surgical procedure, it was valued by some families precisely because it was seen as less barbaric than ECT.[64] It fell into disuse for a combination of reasons and, even more than ECT, became a cultural symbol for a barbaric medical treatment.

The historiography of lobotomy is a study in how the present influences the representation of the past. The first book to provide a well-researched history of psychosurgery was biological psychologist Elliot Valenstein's 1986 *Great and Desperate Cures,* and the depiction there was highly critical.[65] In the 1990s, during the Age of Prozac, and the decade pronounced by George H. W. Bush to be the "decade of the brain," Pressman and Braslow produced accounts that were more balanced, and more sensitive to the context within which lobotomy was seen as cure.[66] More recently, as the excitement about antidepressants that characterized the 1990s has given way to mixed feelings following growing recognition of their limits and adverse effects, Raz has shown that while patients and doctors might have valued the therapeutic powers of lobotomy, it carried serious risks, and Freeman's zealous application was an example of well-intentioned medical overreach.[67] Jenell Johnson's recent study of lobotomy in America recognizes the enthusiasm over positive effects perceived by clinicians, as well as the very considerable public demand that has had no space in social memory.[68] Johnson also shows clearly, however, in ways that Pressman de-emphasized, that the categories of therapy and control were deeply intertwined in lobotomy's use. Freeman was quite open about wanting to promote docility in difficult people, and openly made the case for sacrificing creativity and even dignity in exchange for social adaptability.[69]

All of these therapies developed in the first half of the twentieth century appeared effective—even the clinicians who were most hostile to these forms of treatments conceded that they worked.[70] None of the treatments, however, actually cured mental illnesses—which is also the case with contemporary treatments for mental illness. At best, they provided control and relief for symptoms, but this relief was most welcome. While many patients may have feared the early somatic treatments, there is no question that many also welcomed the symptom relief. Even lobotomy was sought after by patients and their families.[71] And while all the somatic treatments had skeptics in the psychiatric profession, many physicians celebrated new methods with something like euphoria in their early years, reflecting the eagerness to develop cures for stubborn illnesses in an era in which asylum care was in crisis.

The clinical enthusiasm for these treatments came with a cost. Although recent historiography has successfully challenged stereotypes of early somatic treatments as uniformly abusive, all of them had serious side effects—which is why, with the exception of ECT, they have all been phased out. For example, Jack Pressman's work has shown why, in its context, lobotomy was used and valued, but there is also little question in retrospect that it was used excessively, and with too little reflection on what the long-term effects might be. The side effects of these treatments became all the more intolerable once psychopharmaceuticals were developed in the 1950s, providing psychiatrists with what seemed to be dramatically safer alternatives. The history of psychopharmacology, however, has itself been marked by euphoric professional excitement, and early inattention to side effects. Amphetamine can claim to be the first specific medication for a mood disorder, but while it was first developed and marketed in the 1920s, it was not until the 1950s that its addictiveness was recognized by clinicians.[72] Psychiatry was also slow to recognize the evidence that tardive dyskinesia, a movement disorder, was a common side effect of the first generation of antipsychotic medications.[73] There has been similar disregard for adverse effects from antidepressants.[74] Too often, the psychiatric profession has focused narrowly on symptom relief, rather than the overall well-being of patients—although to be fair, psychiatry may in fact be more attentive to patients' overall well-being than many medical specialties.

ECT is the only major somatic treatment developed before the major psychopharmaceuticals that has survived. Although ECT use declined in the 1960s and 1970s, it was revived again in the early 1980s.[75] Interpretations of ECT's revival are, like most interpretations of ECT's history, deeply divided. ECT opponents see contemporary ECT use as a bizarre remnant, and point to its origins in fascist Italy and its initial use on an unwilling patient as evidence for its malevolence. ECT proponents see its survival past the grim years of its early practice as evidence of its inherent utility.[76]

ECT Begins

Ugo Cerletti's work was spurred by a set of developments throughout the world psychiatric community. One was the overcrowding in mental hospitals.[77] Admission of patients was well outpacing discharges. Therapeutic pessimism was abating somewhat with some advances in basic brain science.[78] And the new somatic therapies, for all their faults, also encouraged psychiatrists to think that cases once thought to be hopeless could be helped. But there was little doubt about their faults. The chemical shock therapies were considered dangerous by many psychiatrists, and certainly feared by patients. Chemical convulsive therapy, as developed by Meduna, was most definitely considered effective by psychiatrists, but the fear patients experienced in the beginning of the treatment was a serious drawback. In Italy, home of the famous advances in electricity made by Galvani and Volta, and the neurological advances made by Camille Golgi, Cerletti tried to see if electricity could treat severe mental illness more safely and less fearsomely.

The origin of ECT is worth taking a close look at, because while it is an obscure episode in medical history to people unconcerned with ECT, for people concerned, it has a mythical status. The context of the invention, the clinical rationale for it, and the details of the trial with the first ECT patient are all freighted with meaning. It will not surprise you, if you have read this far, that these aspects of the origin of ECT are understood in radically different ways. It would not be exactly accurate to say that the story is subject to debate, as "debate" implies that there are clearly articulated differences about what happened, or the meaning of what happened. Few, if any, of the facts of this episode are in dispute. Their meaning is, but the dispute has had more the quality of a tacit struggle over emphasis, than a formal debate.

While he was a student, Cerletti visited Germany, and absorbed the influence of Emil Kraepelin, the most important figure in the development of the modern psychiatric diagnosis. In 1935, Cerletti became director of a university psychiatric clinic in Rome, and set up a separate clinic dedicated to the study and practice of Sakel and Meduna's techniques. A year before the first ECT, students of his gave research papers on insulin coma therapy.[79] He rejected the different clinical rationales offered for their treatments by Sakel and Meduna themselves, and argued in a research paper that they worked by a mechanism similar to, but more humane than, lobotomy, destroying neurons and synapses that cause psychotic symptoms. Cerletti and his associates regarded Metrazol as the superior treatment primarily because it was considered cheaper and safer than insulin coma therapy.[80] Their hope was to continue this progress by introducing a means of inducing convulsions that would be still safer and more economical. Yet Cerletti would later assert that ECT was not simply a variant of these treatments, but had a different method of action.

The hypothesis that electricity could safely induce convulsions came from animal observations. Cerletti's associate Lucio Bini observed that in slaughterhouses, shocks given to pigs, in order to stun them before slaughter, would cause convulsions.[81] Initial studies with dogs produced fatalities, because the current passed through the anus, causing cardiac arrest. Purely cranial applications of the electricity were not fatal.[82] They tried the method on a human subject. There were still reservations, though. In the late 1950s, Cerletti told psychiatrist David Impastato, who would have a key role in the introduction of ECT to the United States after its invention in Italy, that the other members of his research team were fearful of applying the electric current. Some worried that it might cause death, permanent brain damage, or "epileptic states." This last concern may seem odd, as the point of the therapy was to induce convulsions, although perhaps the concern was the states would be ongoing.[83] According to this account, then, Cerletti had to overcome these fears to move the research forward. From our perspective, in an era that more highly values restraint in human subjects research, the caution of the associates may seem more desirable. In representing the context this way to Impastato, Cerletti was tapping into an ethos that idolized intrepid medical researchers, who were willing to take risks with patients in the service of general welfare.[84] In Impastato's telling, Cerletti became convinced that there was a vast difference between an amount of current sufficient to induce convulsion and a fatal dose, and "this was his decision and no one else had anything to do with this aspect of the procedure. Cerletti asserts that . . . [ECT] was not an invention but it was merely an audacious act."

Finally, in April 1938, the first human subject was identified. He was a vagrant who had been detained by police in Rome. According to witnesses, he was unable to speak coherently. He could not say his name or provide any other information about himself.[85] Passione, who has done a most careful reconstruction of Cerletti's work and context, says that once the decision to attempt a human trial was made, and a subject identified, Cerletti felt considerable anxiety preceding the attempt, fearing that the patient would die. A member of the team, Luca Alverno, wrote that "[i]n total secrecy, the patient was taken to a remote room on the first floor of the institute. He was quite docile and lay quietly on the examining table. . . . Tension was very high."[86]

In Impastato's account, the first dose of electricity caused only a *petit mal* reaction, after which the patient burst into song.[87] There was, though, cause for anxiety after the initial administration of the shock. The patient uttered what witnesses said was his first coherent sentence since being detained. That coherent sentence was a plea to stop the treatment. But after two shocks, there had been no convulsion, and therefore no treatment, according to the clinical rationale. Impastato continues:

> The Professor suggested that another treatment with a higher voltage be given. The staff objected. Cerletti was apparently prepared to go ahead with it anyway, but the patient said, in clear Italian 'Not again! It will kill me!' This made the Professor think and swallow, but his courage was not lost. He gave the order to proceed at a higher voltage and a longer time: and the first electroconvulsion in man ensued. Thus was born [ECT] out of one man and over the objection of his assistants.[88]

Alverno's account is slightly different:

> Now the question was whether to try again and when to stop before causing any harm. The patient had, up to that point, been relatively unconcerned, but when Cerletti ordered that the voltage and duration be increased for another try, he seemed to realize what was happening and said, 'Careful, the first was pestiferous, the second will be mortiferous.'
> Cerletti gave the signal, and a third impulse produced the usual contractions, followed this time by a grand mal seizure. The patient became

pale, then cyanotic, and stopped breathing. The corneal reflex disappeared, and tachycardia set in. . . . After 45 seconds there was a big stertorous breath, and then the cyanosis disappeared. The pulse became normal, and everybody felt relieved. With a mixture of understatement and optimism Cerletti said simply, 'I can presume that electric current can induce seizures in a man without risks.'[89]

Both witnesses observed clinical success, as the patient's psychotic symptoms remitted, and he became more lucid. This is no more unexpected, based on current clinical science, than his subsequent relapse. According to Alverno, "The first patient improved considerably after the 11 sessions; he regained his memory and his reason, went back to his family in northern Italy, and resumed his work. He also wrote a letter of thanks to Cerletti, but some years later his wife reported that he had begun to suffer from delusions again."[90]

Relapse aside, this first attempt proved to Cerletti that convulsions could be safely induced with electricity with positive results. At this time a therapy that could bring about such a quick remission of symptoms was eagerly sought, and ECT did not require the fearsome loss of consciousness that resulted from insulin coma therapy and Metrazol. Cerletti's team went on with further trials. They reported results to Italy's Higher Institute of Health, claiming that of 36 patients, 11 were cured, 20 showed remarkable improvement, and 5 remained the same.

These numbers might suggest resounding success. Cerletti, though, publicized results diffidently. His first public report was to a limited audience.[91] He was worried by the easiness and cheapness of ECT, fearing it would lead to indiscriminate use, and to overlooking other needs patients had for support.[92] He also developed some theories about why ECT worked that would be largely abandoned in subsequent clinical research. He claimed that the function of the ECT was like an alarm bell, reawakening the patients from their pathological state by placing them violently in front of the "binomial death-life, of which the opposition illness-health represents simply a diminished form." He proposed that ECT led to the formation of a substance in the brain he called "acroaginine," but he never did isolate such a substance.[93]

We often say that judgment of people and events will be left to History. While it is a tempting rhetorical flourish, it is a misleading one. "History" is an abstraction, and does not judge anything. People make historical judgments. The case of Cerletti and the introduction of ECT is a vivid example. There is little dispute over the facts, but judgments vary a lot, depending on people's view of ECT.

Consider the context. ECT was introduced in fascist Italy. But what does the context of ECT's development tell us about it? Leonard Roy Frank is an important critic of ECT, having undergone traumatizing psychiatric treatment in the early 1960s:

My own interest in the subject stems from my having been an involuntary psychiatric inmate for eight months in 1962–1963. Labeled a 'paranoid schizophrenic,' I was forcibly subjected to a course of combined insulin coma-convulsive treatment (50 insulin coma and 35 electroconvulsive treatments) at Twin Pines Hospital in Belmont, California, a peninsula suburb of San Francisco. The procedure resulted in a total and permanent amnesia for the two-year period preceding the last shock treatment.[94]

Frank claims, as many ECT critics have, that ECT is an inherently fascist form of treatment (although there is no evidence anyone on Cerletti's team was fascist). By contrast, two ECT researchers note that its development in such a context, and its subsequent survival, is actually illustrative of its healing power.[95] In other words, rather than tainting it in this account, the treatment's birthplace is all the more evidence of its efficacy, because if it were not effective it would not have survived its unsavory origin. The role of animals in the development of the treatment has also been given different emphases. Bini's observations in the slaughterhouse have been seen by some as evidence of the unsavory origins of ECT; a chapter on ECT in a book critical of psychiatry is entitled "The Slaughterhouse Discovery."[96] By contrast, a sympathetic writer stresses that clinical use on humans was preceded by "painstaking animal trials."[97]

Cerletti's barbarism is sometimes shown by his willingness to proceed with a patient who was begging him to stop, but for Impastato, this intrepid determination was part of what made Cerletti great.[98]

ECT proponents have sometimes pointed to its origins as "hypothesis-driven," as evidence of its scientific pedigree.[99] This matters because psychiatry, often stigmatized within biomedicine as less than scientific anyway, has a history of accidental progress.[100] And the development of ECT was hypothesis driven, in two ways: first by Meduna's hypothesis that induced seizures might cause psychosis to remit, and by Cerletti and Bini's hypothesis that electrically induced convulsions might be safer and less hazardous. But there is a double irony to claiming scientific progress on this basis. First of all, Meduna's hypothesis was based on a premise— the alleged antagonism of epilepsy and schizophrenia—that is no longer regarded as correct. Secondly, Meduna's premise concerned a condition, psychosis, which was abandoned early in the history of ECT as a primary indication. If ECT represents medical progress, then it is another example of accidental progress.

As ECT spread rapidly in the United States in the following two decades, there were frequent attempts to link it to the romance of medical progress that suffused the culture. But ECT had a fraught cultural inheritance, conjuring memories not only of scientific advance but of fearsome science. As its use became common, efforts to represent it as a medical marvel akin to penicillin were met with stern resistance, as they are still today.

Notes

1 Mary Shelley, *Frankenstein, or the Modern Prometheus* (New York: Signet Classic, 1965, originally published 1816).
2 Shelley, *Frankenstein*, 98.
3 Susan Lederer, *Frankenstein: Penetrating the Secrets of Nature* (New Brunswick: Rutgers University Press, 2002), 1, 24, and 31.
4 Dwight Codr argues that this gait, which was not a feature of Shelley's novel, was actually related to observations of walking in the context of polio. Dwight Codr, "Arresting Monstrosity: Polio, Frankenstein, and the Horror Film," *PMLA* (March 2014) 171–187.
5 This is the view taken by Kneeland and Warren in *Pushbutton Psychiatry*, which barely mentions the antecedent convulsive therapies.
6 This is the approach taken by ECT provider and advocate Fink, who emphasizes that the therapy grew out of chemical convulsive therapy. Max Fink, *Electroshock: Restoring the Mind* (New York: Oxford University Press, 1999) ch. 10.
7 Iwan Rhys Morus, *Shocking Bodies: Life, Death, and Electricity in Victorian England* (Gloucestershire: The History Press, 2011).
8 Alan Gauld, *Electrotherapy in the United States* (Minneapolis: The Company, 1977), 1.
9 Morus, *Shocking Bodies*, 7–10.
10 Paola Bertucci, "The Electrical Body of Knowledge: Medical Electricity and Experimental Philosophy in the Mid-Eighteenth Century," in Paola Bertucci and Giulano Pancaldi, eds., *Electric Bodies: Episodes in the History of Medical Electricity* (Bologna: Universita di Bologna, 2001), 50.
11 See, for example, Andreas Killen, *Berlin Electropolis: Shock, Nerves, and German Modernity* (Berkeley: University of California Press, 2006), 30.
12 Gauld, *Electrotherapy in the United States*, 6.
13 Oliver Hochadel, "'My Patient Told Me How To Do It': The Practice of Medical Electricity in the German Enlightenment," in Bertucci and Pancaldi, *Electric Bodies*, 74.
14 Iwan Rhys Morus, "Batteries, Bodies and Belts: Making Careers in Victorian Medical Electricity," in Bertucci and Pancaldi, *Electric Bodies*, 209.
15 Morus, *Shocking Bodies*, 23–25.
16 Marco Bresadola, "Early Galvanism as Technique and Medical Practice," in Bertucci and Pancaldi, *Electric Bodies*, 168, 179.
17 Morus, *Shocking Bodies*, 27–28.
18 See Anson Rabinbach, *The Human Motor: Energy, Fatigue, and the Origins of Modernity* (Berkeley: University of California Press, 1992).
19 Morus, *Shocking Bodies*, 76.
20 Morus, *Shocking Bodies*, 34.
21 Morus, *Shocking Bodies*, 18–19.
22 Gauld, *Electrotherapy in the United States*, 1.
23 Gauld, *Electrotherapy in the United States*, 1.
24 James Delbourgo, "Electrical Humanism in North America: Dr. T. Gale's *Electricity, or Ethereal Fire, Considered* (1802) in Historical Context," in Bertucci and Pancaldi, *Electric Bodies*, 127.
25 Thomas P. Hughes, *Networks of Power: Electrification in Western Society, 1880–1930* (Baltimore: The Johns Hopkins University Press, 1983); David Nye, *Electrifying America: Social Meanings of a New Technology* (Cambridge: MIT Press, 1992).
26 Carolyn Thomas de la Pena, *The Body Electric: How Strange Machines Built the Modern American* (New York: New York University Press, 2003), 1.

27 Nye, *Electrifying America*, 1.
28 Nye, *Electrifying America*, 145.
29 Nye, *Electrifying America*, 151.
30 Nye, *Electrifying America*, 155.
31 Gauld, *Electrotherapy*, 17–25; de la Pena, *The Body Electric*, especially ch. 3.
32 On tuberculosis, see de la Pena, *The Body Electric*, 122–123. On cholera, see Charles Rosenberg, *The Cholera Years: The United States in 1832, 1849, and 1866* (2nd edition, Chicago: University of Chicago Press, 1987), 67. Gauld notes that Edison used electricity to treat "gout concretion"; see *Electrotherapy*, 24. On gout, and also epilepsy, strokes, deafness, and blindness, see Oliver Hochadel, "'My Patient Told Me How To Do It,'" 69. On women's use of electrotherapy to remove hair see Rebecca Herzig, "Subjected to the Current: Batteries, Bodies, and the Early History of Electrification in the United States," *Journal of Social History* 41 (Summer 2008) 867–885. On impotence, see de la Pena, *The Body Electric*, ch. 4.
33 See Paul Starr, *The Social Transformation of American Medicine* (New York: Basic Books, 1984).
34 Killen, *Berlin Electropolis*, 1–5.
35 Edward Shorter, *A Historical Dictionary of Psychiatry* (Oxford: Oxford University Press, 2005), 187. Alienist was the contemporary term for psychiatrist.
36 Shorter, *A Historical Dictionary of Psychiatry*, 187.
37 De la Pena, *The Body Electric*, 102.
38 It is interesting to consider that the electric chair was introduced as a more humane and less painful alternative to other methods of execution, although the first time it was used, the convict required two jolts before dying. "According to witnesses, the process appeared neither efficient nor painless, given the smell of his skin burning under the electrodes and the sight of blood flowing from his nose." De la Pena, *The Body Electric*, 102.
39 There is some overlap between this section and my chapter "Somatic Treatments" in Greg Eghigian, ed., *The Routledge History of Madness* (forthcoming).
40 Allen Ginsberg, "Howl," *Collected Poems, 1947–1980* (New York: Harper and Row, 1980), 130.
41 Historians have debated the extent to which reductions in mortality were due to medical interventions or improvements in hygiene and nutrition; see the introduction to Nancy Tomes, *The Gospel of Germs: Men, Women, and the Microbe in American Life* (Cambridge: Harvard University Press, 1998) for an overview of the literature. But there is no question that the improved outcomes contributed to the image of medical progress.
42 Tomes, *The Gospel of Germs*.
43 This development is surveyed, and mostly lamented, in Ian Dowbiggin, *The Quest for Mental Health* (Cambridge: Cambridge University Press, 2011).
44 W.H. Auden, "In Memoriam Sigmund Freud," in *Another Time: Poems* (London: Faber & Faber, 1940), 118.
45 Thomas Szasz, *Coercion as Cure: A Critical History of Psychiatry* (New Brunswick, NJ: Transaction Publishers, 2009).
46 Andrew Scull, "Somatic Treatments and the Historiography of Psychiatry," *History of Psychiatry* V (1994); Joel Braslow, *Mental Ills and Bodily Cures: Psychiatric Treatment in the First Half of the Twentieth Century* (Berkeley: University of California, 1997); Elliot S. Valenstein, *Great and Desperate Cures: The Rise and Decline of Psychosurgery and Other Radical Treatments for Mental Illness* (New York: Basic Books, 1986); Pressman, *Last Resort*; Edward Shorter, *A History of Psychiatry: From the Era of the Asylum to the Age of Prozac* (New York: John Wiley and Sons, 1997); D.B. Doroshow, "Performing a Cure for Schizophrenia: Insulin Coma Therapy on the Wards," *Journal of the History of Medicine and Allied Sciences* 62, 2 (2007) 213–243.

47 See Shorter, *A History of Psychiatry,* a general history of psychiatry that expresses an unabashed preference for the somatic style; Braslow, *Mental Ills and Bodily Cures;* David Healy, *The Anti-Depressant Era* (Cambridge: Harvard University Press, 1997); David Healy, *The Creation of Psychopharmacology* (Cambridge: Cambridge University Press, 2002); Pressman, *Last Resort;* Elliott Valenstein, *Blaming the Brain: The Truth about Drugs and Mental Health* (New York: The Free Press, 1998); Sheldon Gelman, *Medicating Schizophrenia: A History* (New Brunswick: Rutgers University Press, 1999); Jonathan Metzl, *Prozac on the Couch: Prescribing Gender in the Era of Wonder Drugs* (Duke University Press, 2003).

48 See especially Pressman on lobotomy in *Last Resort* and Braslow on a range of therapies in *Mental Ills and Bodily Cures.* The Thompson quote is from *The Making of the English Working Class* (New York: Vintage Books, 1966, originally published 1963), 12: "I am seeking to rescue the poor stockinger, the Luddite cropper, the 'obsolete' hand-loom weaver, the 'utopian' artisan, and even the deluded follower of Joanna Southcott, from the enormous condescension of posterity."

49 See especially Healy's work on psychopharmacology in *The Anti-Depressant Era* and *The Creation of Psychopharmacology.*

50 Andrew Scull, *Madness in Civilization: A Cultural History of Schizophrenia from the Bible to Freud, from the Madhouse to Modern Medicine* (Princeton: Princeton University Press, 2015), 508.

51 This point is effectively developed in Mical Raz's recent *The Lobotomy Letters: The Making of American Psychosurgery* (Rochester: University of Rochester Press, 2013).

52 Nicolas Rasmussen, *On Speed: The Many Lives of Amphetamine* (New York: New York University Press, 2008).

53 On hydrotherapy, see Braslow, *Mental Ills and Bodily Cures,* 38–52.

54 Shorter, *A History of Psychiatry,* 194–194.

55 Scull, *Madness in Civilization,* 302.

56 Shorter, *A History of Psychiatry,* 194.

57 Jenell Johnson, *American Lobotomy: A Rhetorical History* (Ann Arbor: University of Michigan Press, 2014), 29.

58 See, for example, Lothar B. Kalinowsky and Paul H. Hoch, *Shock Treatments and Other Somatic Procedures in Psychiatry* (New York: Grune and Stratton, 1946), one of the most widely used textbooks of the era.

59 On insulin coma therapy in an American hospital, see Doroshow, "Performing a Cure for Schizophrenia."

60 Scull, *Madness in Civilization,* 502.

61 Sylvia Nasar, *A Beautiful Mind: The Life of Mathematical Genius and Nobel Laureate John Nash* (New York: Touchstone, 1998).

62 Nasar, *A Beautiful Mind,* 292–293.

63 Nasar, *A Beautiful Mind,* 250, 306.

64 Braslow, *Mental Ills and Bodily Cures,* 137.

65 Valenstein, *Great and Desperate Cures.*

66 Pressman, *Last Resort;* Braslow, *Mental Ills and Bodily Cures.*

67 Raz, *The Lobotomy Letters.*

68 Johnson, *American Lobotomy.*

69 Johnson, *American Lobotomy,* 30.

70 Psychiatrists oriented toward talking therapies were sometimes relatively hostile to physical treatments—although as I argue in ch. 4, the extent of disagreement between these two major psychiatric styles has sometimes been exaggerated.

71 See Pressman, *Last Resort,* 81, 102, 122–123, for example.

72 Rasmussen, *On Speed,* 55, 143.

73 Gelman, *Medicating Schizophrenia;* see 12–13, for example.

74 David Healy, *Let Them Eat Prozac* (New York: New York University Press, 2004).

75 This decline and rise in usage is difficult to document definitively, because there is no central body that keeps track of ECT usage nationally. The pattern outlined here is mentioned in many impressionistic accounts by practitioners.

76 For example, "That such a seemingly crude and invasive treatment emanating from pre-World War II central Europe should even remain extant is remarkable—and telling." Matthew V. Rudorfer and Frederick K. Goodwin, Introduction to C. Edward Coffey, *The Clinical Science of Electro-Convulsive Therapy* (Washington, D.C.: American Psychiatric Press, Inc., 1993).

77 Roberta Passione, "Electricity and Life, Cerletti's Electroshock and the 'Acro-aginine' Theory," in Bertucci and Pancaldi, *Electric Bodies*, 264–265.

78 Passione points out that Camille Golgi's discoveries of the nature of neurons gave a boost to therapeutic optimism. "Electricity and Life," in Bertucci and Pancaldi, *Electric Bodies*, 264–265.

79 Roberta Passione, "Italian Psychiatry in an International Context: Ugo Cerletti and the Case of Electroshock," *History of Psychiatry* 15, 1 (March 2004) 83–104, 89.

80 Passione, "Italian Psychiatry in an International Context," 88.

81 Luca Alverno, "The Origins of Electroconvulsive Therapy," *Wisconsin Medical Journal* (February 1990) 54–56, 54.

82 Passione, "Italian Psychiatry in an International Context," 89.

83 David J. Impastato, "The Story of the First Electroshock Treatment," *American Journal of Psychiatry* 116 (1959–60) 1112–1114.

84 See Bert Hansen, *Picturing Medical Progress From Pasteur to Polio: A History of Mass Media Images and Popular Attitudes in America* (New Brunswick: Rutgers University Press, 2009).

85 David J. Impastato, "The Story of the First Electroshock Treatment."

86 Alverno, "The Origins of Electroconvulsive Therapy," 54.

87 David J. Impastato, "The Story of the First Electroshock Treatment," 1113.

88 Impastato, "The Story of the First Electroshock Treatment," 1114.

89 Alverno, "The Origins of Electroconvulsive Therapy," 55.

90 Alverno, "The Origins of Electroconvulsive Therapy," 55.

91 Passione, "Electricity and Life," in Bertucci and Pancaldi, *Electric Bodies*, 274.

92 Passione, "Italian Psychiatry in an International Context," 90–91.

93 Passione, "Electricity and Life," in Bertucci and Pancaldi, *Electric Bodies*, 280.

94 Leonard Roy Frank, *The History of Shock Treatment* (San Francisco: Leonard Roy Frank, 1978) ix.

95 Introduction by Rudorfer. Goodwin in Coffey, *The Clinical Science of Electro-Convulsive Therapy*, xvii.

96 Joseph Berke, *I Haven't Had to Go Mad Here* (Harmondsworth: Penguin Books, 1979, originally published as *Butterfly Man*, 1977).

97 Burns, "The Scientific Origins of Electroconvulsive Therapy: A Conceptual History."

98 Impastato, "The Story of the First Electroshock Treatment," 1114.

99 Introduction by Rudorfer and Goodwin to Coffey, *The Clinical Science of Electro-Convulsive Therapy*, xvii; Shorter and Healy, *Shock Therapy*, 22.

100 The discovery of the psychiatric benefits of both early antidepressants and antipsychotics were accidental developments from their trials for other illnesses, for example.

2   Trying to Make Progress

"Hope for Tired Minds"

Throughout the history of ECT, patients have both attested to damage it has done, and expressed gratitude for the relief and hope it can provide. In the mid-1940s, when ECT was a new treatment, a patient named Frank Kimball wrote about as definite an endorsement as one will find from a patient of any therapy.[1] His account uses the word "miracle," perhaps the single word most laden with the optimistic expectations of medicine that became such a potent cultural force in the mid-twentieth century. Kimball was a patient at Boston's famous McLean Hospital in the 1930s and 1940s.[2] He had held a number of different jobs after college, teaching high school and working in insurance and investments, and he became a trustee of Boston University. Then he went into politics, which he later decided was inappropriate for his personality type. He said his illness was due to overwork and anxiety, and a rejection by his town of a plan for a World War memorial park he and a committee had proposed. He began to suffer from insomnia, "as night after night my mental wheels ground out schemes and churned over my mistakes, real and imaginary." This culminated in a crisis leading to hospitalization at Channing Sanitarium in Wellesley in 1927. His chart from his admission described him as

> retarded in speech and action; shaky; underweight; self-accusatory; afraid of arrest for misuse of funds; suspicious of nurses, believing them to be detectives; obsessed with fears of business failure and showing increasing aversion toward family and friends.

He was transferred to McLean in 1931, where he did some occupational therapy but described little interest in people or activities, except for a mild interest in reading. Although depressed mood was his primary complaint, he also had delusions, believing that sounds in nature, doors, and floor-boards were forming sentences, speaking to him. In one episode during his hospitalization, he had a delusion that he was visiting home. He ate all the oranges his wife had prepared for breakfast, and then snuck out. In his view, the efforts of the staff at McLean kept him from the worst of despair, but he got no better.

No better, that is, until one of them suggested ECT. In 1942, when he was 70 years old and had been ill for at least 15 years, in his words, ECT "wrought a miracle!" After a short course of ECT, he left the hospital and rejoined his family. He was released in March 1943, about which he wrote "I was free! Free! At last, and well." He went home, he said, not only to normal life, but to a life "far better even than that of my first half-century of normal living." After his discharge, acquaintances described him as being like his old self, and long-standing social phobias faded. Pleasure in activities he had enjoyed before his illness, like music, churchgoing, time with family, and travel, returned. There is no description of pain during the treatment; rather, he cheerfully related amnesia of the treatment. And that amnesia is the only memory loss he recorded.

The history of ECT contains a lot of evidence that is inconvenient for partisans on different sides of the controversy. When one side accuses the other of cherry-picking the data, the accusation is often correct. Sometimes this selectiveness can be a matter of not reading or citing testimony that would complicate the case. Other times, it is a matter of acknowledging complicating evidence, but ignoring or dismissing its significance.[3] Kimball's account is a case of the former. Although it is not buried in an obscure archive, but in a magazine article easily available from libraries, you will not find a reference to it in attacks on ECT practice.

The development of ECT in Italy in the 1930s was a deliberate attempt to make scientific and medical progress—to build on the first clinical successes in treating severe and chronic mental illnesses, and to develop a therapy that would be safer and less frightening than others that were available. As the use of ECT spread in American psychiatry during the 1940s and 1950s, its promoters saw it in these terms, and some undoubtedly hoped its image would be something like the miracle cure that Kimball described. This was an era of medical heroism. Historian Bert Hansen has documented the ways medical advances—some of them by this time many decades old, such as Pasteur's development of a vaccine for rabies—were, starting in the 1940s, being celebrated in various media, including novels, movies, advertisements, and comic books.[4] The brave and tireless medical researcher was becoming an iconic figure, and an emblem of the excitement medical advance was generating.

For the most part, the new psychiatric somatic treatments did not generate this popular excitement. Freudian therapy did, and later, the tranquilizer Miltown would.[5] Cerletti was mostly unknown to the lay public; he was no Pasteur. ECT's promoters had only uneven success in creating an aura of progress for ECT, even among their professional colleagues. ECT use certainly spread rapidly in American psychiatry, and many practitioners were clearly persuaded of its utility. Yet the most enthusiastic clinical writings on ECT often contained a note of defensiveness even in these early years, a sign that promoters felt the need to persuade skeptical colleagues. Patients, too, had apprehensions. Well before the publication of *One Flew Over the Cuckoo's Nest* and other Hollywood movies that psychiatrists would later blame for making their patients afraid of ECT, there are signs in the very early years of patient fear. Another account from the mid-1940s tells the story of a psychology student who had himself helped to administer ECT before showing signs of mania and depression, leading to his own treatment.[6] His anxiety was so great during the prepping that he was sweating profusely. This was described as common for patients about to have ECT. The patient later felt that he recovered from his illness, although he credited that more to his relationship to his doctor than to the ECT.

Historians of medicine have, in recent decades, worked hard to dislodge naïve or heroic notions of medical progress, and to move medical history away from a preoccupation with great doctors.[7] This work has had salutary effects. It has spawned more critical history, and opened up the history of medicine beyond clinicians to the study of all affected by sickness and medicine—that is, everyone. If these efforts have had a downside, it is that the critique of progress narratives has become an instant reflex. I will argue in the conclusion that while historians need to think critically about what constitutes progress, we also should think carefully about whether we want to do away with the concept altogether. In any event, my goal in this chapter is slightly different. I am not attempting to add to the critique of progress narratives, nor am I trying to resurrect them. Rather, I want to show how the idea of medical progress "worked" as part of the history itself. How did the idea of medical progress function in the consciousness of the doctors who brought ECT into American medical practice? What were its limits?

ECT Comes to America

The introduction and spread of ECT in the United States was accomplished by a combination of émigré psychiatrists and natives. The key émigré figures were part of Cerletti's team in Italy. One was Lothar Kalinowsky, who was originally from Berlin. As a student in Germany, he had the opportunity to hear lectures by Emil Kraepelin, often considered the foundational figure in the development of the biological model of mental illness; Kalinowsky found the lectures extremely dull.[8] Kalinowsky had actually hoped to be a pathologist, and only became a psychiatrist because a position was available in the early 1920s, when the German inflation made having a job essential.[9] He also studied in Vienna with Wagner von Jauregg, the inventor of malaria fever therapy, before moving back to Berlin.[10] Kalinowsky's mother was Jewish, and he lost his hospital position due to the Nazi rise to power. He moved to Rome in 1933.[11] He was present when Cerletti treated the first ECT patient.[12] He thus had unusually rich direct exposure to the main innovators in somatic psychiatry of his era. The pact between Hitler and Mussolini forced him to leave Italy for the United States near the beginning of World War II, but he stopped first in France, Holland, and England, and introduced ECT in each of those countries.[13] In early publications on ECT, he touted the treatment as solving all the problems associated with chemical convulsive therapy, claiming that it removed all the dread patients had of the treatment.[14] It can be hard to appreciate this now, when ECT has become a symbol for fear of medicine, but this is one of the commonest themes in the early clinical literature. As Kalinowsky put it in *The Lancet,* "All the disagreeable subjective sensations present in Cardiazol [Metrazol] therapy are missing."[15] He wanted to settle in the United Kingdom, but was unable to find a job there,[16] so he moved to the United States, where Adolf Meyer helped him to obtain an appointment at the New York State Psychiatric Institute under Nolan Lewis. He became the leading exponent and authority for ECT in North America in the early decades of its use.

Another émigré from Cerletti's team was Renato Almansi, an Italian Jew who came directly to the United States, actually carrying an ECT machine with him. Almansi initially had trouble finding interested psychiatrists to work with him, having tried with the heads of psychiatry departments in Philadelphia, Boston, and New York. He eventually formed a collaboration with Impastato, who had relocated to Manhattan.[17] Kalinowsky arrived in New York shortly afterward, and began working with Almansi and Impastato at Columbus Hospital, later becoming associated with the New York Psychiatric Institute, where he began administering ECT in summer 1940.[18]

There is uncertainty about who first performed ECT in the United States. There were early ECTs performed close in time in New York, Chicago, Boston, Philadelphia, and Cincinnati. Some have claimed to know which was first, but I believe a careful scrutiny of the primary source material shows the exact chronology to be hard to determine. Certainly some of the doctors who did early ECTs were eager to claim priority, however much ECT's detractors might see this as a dubious honor. These sources are more useful for what they yield about how early American ECT was perceived, depicted, and disseminated, than for establishing primacy.

In the late 1950s, after nearly two decades of ECT use in America, a Philadelphia physician named Sidney Pulver learned of a rumor that a patient at the Institute of the Pennsylvania Hospital had been the first American ECT patient.[19] The rumor stoked his curiosity. After some inquiry, Pulver believed that the first American ECT was performed by a Chicago neurologist named Victor Gonda.[20] Gonda was himself an immigrant, originally trained in Budapest early in the twentieth century.[21] He served as a sanitarium psychiatrist during World War I, where he treated "shell shocked" patients.[22] He emigrated to the United States in 1924, and became an attending neurologist at Cook County Hospital and a professor at Loyola School of Medicine.[23] He was familiar with chemical convulsive therapy, and developed a close relationship with Meduna. Gonda had also been corresponding with Cerletti, and had an ECT machine imported from Genoa in 1939. Gonda first tried the machine on animals, producing convulsions. He also tried the machine on his own thigh and hit his leg on a table, rendering himself unable to walk for a few days.[24] He gave the first treatment to a patient in January 1940 in Chicago's Parkway Sanitarium. His son recalled

> the anxieties and the tensions [his father] experienced with the giving of the first few treatments, having accompanied . . . [him] to the Sanitarium on these occasions. By May of 1940, dad had treated several patients and had learned many nuances relative to the treatment.[25]

Gonda's own published report came out the next year, and stressed the ways ECT was an advance over Metrazol.[26] Bone injuries were less common because the seizure was less violent. Patients who used to vomit after Metrazol convulsions did not vomit after ECT. There never seemed to be an unplanned second convulsion, as would happen sometimes with Metrazol. The care after the convulsion was easier, because the recovery was quicker. Above all, Gonda—like virtually every other early ECT practitioner—was struck by the reduction in fear and resistance from patients. His description of one patient experience is especially powerful:

> I have now under treatment a patient suffering from paranoid type of schizophrenia who, undergoing metrazol . . . and insulin therapy, objected bitterly to the continuation of the insulin treatment. Without his being aware of it, I initiated electric treatments. Signs of improvement soon set in. One morning he begged me to put the electrodes on his head more frequently, because, as he said, on the days that I did this he felt much better all day.[27]

Gonda further claimed that "not one patient thus far objected to the continuation of the treatment."[28] The reduced discomfort and fear from patients also meant that fewer assistants were needed, because there was no need to subdue a struggling patient. The head pain from the electricity was not perceived because of the rapid loss of consciousness. Gonda knew well that it would have been painful otherwise because, as he said, "The current is very painful. I convinced myself of this by applying it to my thigh."[29]

By the time he wrote this article, Gonda had treated 40 patients. Of these, 29 had schizophrenia; 58.6% showed complete remission, 20.7% were improved, and 20.7% were not improved. Three patients with involutional (age-related) psychosis were, he said, completely better. Of eight "depressive cases," seven were recovered. The other, who had been ill for six years previously, was unimproved. The seven who recovered had relapses after leaving the hospital. Combining his observations with other published reports from the time, he found remission results at least as good as those from Metrazol, but with fewer problems. He concluded by strongly emphasizing a need for psychotherapy afterwards, considering this equal in importance to the convulsion itself.

Clarence Neymann, also of Cook County Hospital, also adopted ECT use early. Neymann's first publication came out in November 1943.[30] At the time of writing, hundreds of patients had been treated at the hospital. Although Neymann found ECT (and precursor shock treatments) to be effective, his article dissented from some glowing clinical reports of the time. He wrote, "The reports of the instantaneous results of shock therapy, and especially of electric shock therapy, are often ridiculous,"[31] adding that if he wanted to be rash, he could say all his patients improved, but only if he were to leave out any accounting of just how many days they were well. Neymann was one of the first to draw attention to the strong possibility of relapse, and he also urged psychotherapy or psychoanalysis following shock treatment in order to increase the chances of recovery. He stands out as a voice of caution, and while he clearly believed that ECT was worth using, he did not think its true value would be clear for another 10 years.

According to Pulver, Impastato and Almansi had used the machine that Almansi had brought from Italy to begin treating patients at Columbus Hospital in New York in February 1940. This would make Gonda's use the first, by one month.[32] Pulver had this on good authority, as he had received a letter from Impastato himself saying that he had treated his first ECT patient then.[33] But Impastato's notes on his first ECT patient, housed in the archives of the American Psychiatric Association (APA), seem to show that Impastato remembered incorrectly, as they indicate that his patient received her first ECT treatment on January 7, 1940.[34]

The APA archives contain case notes on Impastato and Almansi's first patient, a 29-year-old Manhattan woman. She was engaged in paranoid and self-destructive behavior, according to Impastato's notes on examining her in December 1939:

> Says she has been ill 8 years. Started by refusing to eat & then began to say that people wanted to take her head off etc. She was at Central Islip & she came out 6 years ago. She has been the same since. Stays by herself—doesn't go out, doesn't talk to anyone, complain of headache, talk to herself, at time [illegible word] angry has not broken anything but has been mildly assaultive. Imagines people are against her etc.[35]

Her ECT treatments continued over the course of the year. In October, Impastato wrote, "She used to talk like a machine. Now she is nice and quiet." In 1944, the patient having evidently been released some time before, Impastato contacted her and requested a follow-up visit to see how she was doing. Her father came in and reported that she had gained weight and was quieter, but still did not talk "normally," and was unable to work but did help with housework. There must have been limits to any clinical improvement she showed, however. In 1945, under circumstances that are not clear, she was re-admitted to Central Islip. Impastato contacted the institution on behalf of the family, who wanted her released. He said that she had been in his care the previous years, that she had been improving with ECT, and that the family was capable of caring for her. Two years later, he needed to write a similar letter to Manhattan State Hospital, asking for her early "parole." He received a response from a physician at the hospital saying that she showed "signs of advanced schizophrenic deterioration," and was "actively responding to hallucinations, peculiarly behaved, untidy in her appearance, incontinent of urine, and has to be urged to attend to her personal needs" and was therefore unfit to be released to the care of her relatives. In 1957, she had a lobotomy, possibly because of some "assaultive and destructive" behavior Impastato referred to while testifying to her eligibility for disability payments that year.

A Boston team also adopted ECT early, possibly contemporaneously or even before Impastato.[36] Boston psychiatrist Isadore Green learned of the development of ECT in Italy by reading about it in an Italian journal. Cerletti's first publications on ECT contained no details about how to construct an ECT machine. Green, physiotherapist Louis Feldman, and electrical engineer F. T. Davis constructed their own machine, and tested it on rabbits. These tests went on for six months, and a pathologist examined the brains of the rabbits, determining that there was no lasting brain damage. They were not allowed to do ECT at Boston State Hospital, but were "harbored" by Eliza Lindberg of the Bosworth Hospital in Brookline. At the first ECT they performed, "when the button was pressed everybody looked the other way." Green claimed in a 1969 letter to Impastato that they gave their first treatment "on or about January 1939," a full year before Impastato and Almansi. Impastato—straining a little to insist on his own priority, I think—cited their first published report, from the 1941 *New England Journal of Medicine,* and claimed that it cited only foreign sources. Impastato reasoned that if Green and his colleagues had treated patients earlier, then they would have cited their own experience. But he either did not read the entire paper or forgot it, because while the paper cites foreign research on the first page, it focuses entirely on their own clinical work in the remainder.[37]

The first author on this paper was prominent Boston psychiatrist Abraham Myerson, a well-known expert on depression who was involved in developing drug treatments. According to Green, Myerson was initially dubious about ECT, but later joined Green's ECT team.[38] Myerson became a vigorous advocate of ECT, touring New England to spread word of his views that it offered fast remission and was harmless.[39] In their *New England Journal of Medicine* article, Myerson, Green, and Feldman stressed how ECT was an advance over chemical treatments because it was easier to administer, and more palatable to unwilling patients. "Although no shock therapy can be classed as pleasant, electric shock therapy is the least disturbing to the patient and creates less fear and resistance to the treatment."[40] They touted ECT's "reasonable safety," saying that injuries were rare if it was done carefully, and that the general bodily reaction was less disturbing than with Metrazol. This article was also important for being one of the first to cite better results with affective problems—Myerson's interest—than with psychosis. They said it was of "unequaled value" in depressive states,[41] and went so far as to say that schizophrenia, the illness for which ECT was first developed, was not an indication, except in catatonic cases. They explained that in schizophrenia, some delusions could be dispelled by the treatment but that "the retreat and the incapacity to meet the situations in life were only transitorily changed for the better."[42]

There was also early ECT use in Philadelphia. An assistant of Bini's was passing through the city in the fall of 1939, bringing the new therapy to the attention of Joseph Hughes, an electrophysiologist, who designed his own machine.[43] In their first publication on the subject, Hughes's team claimed to be the first Americans to try it, but they treated their first human patient in May 1940 and were likely not the first.[44] They had also experimented on animals and noted that cats not only responded with convulsions but "showed no memory of the experience," evidenced by the continued friendliness of the cats.[45] Although they found some possibility of side effects, including fractures, the thrust of their article was the better results with ECT as compared to chemical shock treatments.

Other cities with relatively early ECT practice included Cincinnati, where doctors began use in April 1941, and Washington, D.C., where famed lobotomist Walter Freeman invited Impastato and Almansi to demonstrate in December 1940.[46] By the end of 1940, the American companies Rahm and Lectra were already producing ECT machines.[47] Almansi and Impastato reported in September 1940 that ECT had by that time been introduced to Germany and England as well, and that "thousands of convulsions" had been induced.[48] In this paper, which Impastato would later claim was the first American publication on ECT,[49] they emphasized the ways it improved on Metrazol. They said that the complete unconscious state ECT produces meant patients would have no memory of the treatment, and therefore no resistance to it in the future. They also said that, unlike with Metrazol, "there is no postconvulsive excitement, or when it is present it is very mild."[50]

Their readers would at this time have had experience with Metrazol, but little if any with ECT. This was ECT in its most primitive state, without muscle relaxants or anesthesia, and their description is worth paying close attention to:

> The machine is supplied by the ordinary alternating house current of 110 volts. It contains two circuits: a direct to measure the resistance of the patient's head, and an alternating to produce the convulsion. A change-over switch selects the current desired. The electrodes consist of silver ribbons mounted on rubber pads. These are in turn mounted on metallic tongs which allow an easy application of the electrodes to the patient's head. The convulsive threshold for each patient is determined by beginning with low voltages, usually 60 volts, for one-tenth of a second. If this fails to produce a convulsion, a second attempt with slightly higher voltage can be made fifteen to thirty minutes later. In most cases convulsions will occur with 80 volts.

The spell follows immediately after the current has been applied, or after a latent period of a few seconds to about thirty seconds. There is usually a cry, which is followed by a tonic phase lasting from twenty to thirty seconds, at the end of which there is a brief interval of apnea. . . . Usually there is no voidance of urine or feces. The patient now goes into a deep stupor which lasts about five minutes. Then follows a period of confusion which lasts from five to ten minutes, at the end of which time the patient is usually clear, but has no recollection of the treatment. The treatments are given two or three times a week, and a full course consists of thirty sessions. If the patient is going to improve, this will manifest itself usually before the tenth treatment.[51]

They described some safety precautions taken before the treatment. These included ruling out organic diseases of the cardiovascular or nervous systems and barring from treatment anyone over age 50. They concluded by saying that electroencephalogram results were similar to those obtained after Metrazol, but milder, and that they had induced 100 convulsions without any complications. They did not feel they could confidently evaluate their success with this small database. They were, however, very active in disseminating the treatment, lecturing, publishing, and giving demonstrations live or on film.[52]

By 1941—three years after the first attempted ECT treatment—42% of mental hospitals in the United States had ECT machines in use.[53] In New York State, by 1943 all but three of the state hospitals were using ECT.[54] ECT came to be used in all industrialized countries, and was adopted in mental hospitals in the developing world as well. This might seem like a fast spread for a therapy that had not been subject to much testing. But hospital personnel were eager to try anything for many of their chronic patients; Healy notes that in the 1950s "the use of chlorpromazine (Thorazine) spread like wildfire through American asylums,"[55] and Pressman stresses that this was one reason for the widespread use of lobotomy. Another reason for the spread of ECT was that although first developed for schizophrenia, ECT proved most useful for mood disorders such as mania and depression, which quickly became the primary indications.[56] Perhaps most importantly, when ECT was introduced, clinicians viewed it more as a technical modification of an existing treatment, convulsive therapy, in which Metrazol was replaced by the application of electricity. Many doctors continued to use both insulin coma and Metrazol alongside ECT for years.

An early American textbook on ECT and the other shock treatments for clinicians was *Shock Treatment in Psychiatry: A Manual* by Lucie Jessner and V. Gerard Ryan, which appeared in 1941.[57] Although this manual continued to recommend insulin coma and Metrazol for patients with severe mental illnesses, the dominant theme in this book is the dramatic progress represented by ECT. The first two sections review the clinical science of insulin coma and Metrazol, describing clinical benefits, but also dwelling at length on the risks, discomfort, and fear, as well as mediocre remission rates, well under 50%, that made them perhaps better than no treatment at all but hardly miracle cures. The concluding section on ECT is rife with intimations of progress: a less violent fit than with Metrazol, less fear on the part of the patient because of the quick descent into unconsciousness and the amnesia of the treatment, and better remission rates. This was not a breathless account of a perfect therapy, though. ECT was very new, and the authors were careful not to make premature claims. Also, at this point ECT was being performed without anesthesia or muscle relaxants. Bone fractures, they said, could be avoided by removal of dentures, a mouth gag, a hard mattress, hyperextension of the dorsal spine, and lots of assistants. In an introduction to the book, the psychiatrist Harry Solomon wrote: "'Shock therapy' has thrust its non-too-pretty form into the field of psychiatry. Whatever the process of producing 'shock,' the process itself is distasteful."[58] Jessner and Ryan also emphasized that all three therapies should be used as preludes to psychotherapy, as measures that could restore the patient's engagement with the world so that psychotherapeutic work could commence.

The major textbook on the shock therapies of the era, though, was published five years later by Kalinowsky and Paul Hoch.[59] Hoch was also an immigrant, born in Budapest in 1902. He studied medicine in Switzerland and Germany before coming to the United States.[60] After his immigration to the United States, he directed a shock treatment unit in Manhattan State Hospital, which took up insulin coma, Metrazol, and ECT as each one was introduced. In 1943, he joined the New York State Psychiatric Institute. He later became New York State's Commissioner of Mental Hygiene, a position he held from 1955 to 1964.[61] His main clinical interest was schizophrenia.[62]

After Hoch's death, numerous tributes were published in professional journals. Colleagues remembered him warmly as a talented administrator, and a vigorous advocate for cautious empirical research on new therapies over faddish enthusiasm, and one who favored somatic treatments but respected psychoanalysts.[63] He was among the first psychiatrists in America to try the antipsychotic medications when they became available, and he had an interest in the therapeutic possibilities of psychedelic drugs.[64] His legacy, though, is tainted by his involvement in conducting CIA- and Army-sponsored experiments with psychedelic drugs on human subjects without consent. The most publicized case involved professional tennis player Harold Blauer, who sought psychiatric treatment for depression, was given psychedelic drugs without his knowledge, and unexpectedly died. Hoch was a P.I. on the study. The Army admitted culpability some years afterwards and Blauer's family received a settlement.[65]

Kalinowsky and Hoch's book, published in America in 1946, just eight years after the first ECT in Italy, discussed insulin coma, Metrazol, and ECT. It went through four editions, and was the standard work on somatic therapies in psychiatry for more than 30 years.[66] All three therapies discussed in the book were described as "shock treatments," but the authors distinguished insulin coma therapy from the other two, arguing that although convulsions could be present in insulin coma, they were not the therapeutic mechanism that they were for the other two.[67] This usage of the term "shock treatment" was common in psychiatry in this era, although a few authors used the term to encompass some other somatic treatments, such as malaria fever therapy and prolonged sleep therapy. Although there is some evidence that Cerletti thought ECT was a new treatment, with a different therapeutic basis from chemical convulsive therapy, Kalinowsky and Hoch did not. This helped set the tone for the consistent belief of American clinicians that ECT was a technical modification to chemical convulsive therapy, and not a new therapy.[68]

The advantages clinicians saw in ECT were not thought to eliminate problems with compliance. There would continue to be patients who resisted the treatment, although doctors thought these would be mostly patients who had previous experience with Metrazol.[69] They recommended drugging reluctant patients with sedatives, which could also be used to calm patients who were "restless, whining, or panicky" after ECT.[70]

Kalinowsky and Hoch also firmly asserted that ECT was safe. Damage to the bones and physical pain could be managed by muscle relaxants and anesthesia. There were some side effects, at least to some patients, they conceded. They described the aftermath of ECT for some patients in a passage that sounds like it could have come from one of the newly popular superhero comic books of the time that described powerful but dangerous powers developing after exposure to new technologies. After convulsions, Kalinowsky and Hoch explained,

> some patients, particularly males, become dangerously assaultive, develop enormous strength, try to escape, run around and injure themselves, and may strike anyone who tries to control them. . . . It seems to be more frequent in patients who have a strong fear of the treatment. Treatment of this reaction is prophylactic; its recurrence may be prevented by intravenous injection of sodium amytal immediately prior to treatment.[71]

They denied any likelihood of lasting intellectual impairment, and claimed that patients who complained tended to be neurotic or hypochondriacal.[72] They argued that clinical reports of amnesia were only confirming what everyone agreed on, that there is some short-term memory loss. The issue of memory loss will be explored more in Chapter Six, but note that they did not have strong grounds for this confidence, as there were few studies of the cognitive effects of ECT at that time. Despite their confidence, cognitive impairment was, anyway, the one area they thought Metrazol had some advantage.[73] And, while they acknowledged some risk of impairment, they also included a reminder that sometimes medical treatments, such as surgeries, are just risky, and medical treatment sometimes necessitates risk.[74] The passages on ECT's safety show some defensiveness, a need to persuade skeptics. Kalinowsky's enthusiasm for ECT was such that, in the early years of unmodified ECT, he could at once concede at least some risk of bone fractures and still refer to the therapy as essentially harmless.[75] This is not simply a measure of his regard for the therapy, though. It speaks also to a higher threshold for adverse effects in medicine at that time, to the vast perceived improvements in comfort ECT provided over Metrazol, and to the desperation patients and doctors felt responding to severe mental illness in the era before antipsychotic and antidepressant medications.

The risk of fracture was reduced by the introduction of curare into convulsive therapy by American physician A. E. Bennett.[76] Curare is a naturally occurring substance that causes muscle paralysis. After working with it on a number of patients, he concluded that it would make fractures from the treatment virtually impossible in the absence of pre-existing bone pathology. Because curare could be scarce, he also experimented with synthetic substitutes, which came to be the norm in ECT treatment. By the 1950s, modified ECT, with the use of both muscle relaxants and anesthesia, was not universal in American psychiatry, but it was the standard of care.[77]

ECT's early years were also marked by another major shift in clinical practice, in the primary indications. Developed for schizophrenia on the basis of Meduna's hypothesis on the inverse relation with epilepsy, ECT was quickly noticed to be more effective for affective disorders, particularly bipolar disorder (known as manic depression at that time) and severe depression. There had been observations of the greater efficacy for affective disorders for Metrazol as well.[78] And most clinical observers found the convulsive therapies to be no better for psychoses than insulin coma therapy.[79] Malzberg's survey actually found insulin coma to be superior to convulsive therapy for psychosis.[80] But there were numerous observations of ECT's better efficacy for affective disorders in the early 1940s.[81] ECT would continue to be used for a very wide range of mental disorders, including psychoses, at least into the 1960s. Particularly because the precise reason convulsive therapies were therapeutic remained obscure, it was natural for clinicians to try them for other intractable illnesses, even as the evidence mounted that they were most powerful for mood disorders.

The early shift to affective disorders as the primary indication for convulsive therapies actually deepened the mystery of how the therapies worked. If the original rationale for inducing convulsions was the supposed inverse relationship between epilepsy and schizophrenia, and there was no supposition of such a relationship between epilepsy and affective disorders, why did ECT produce therapeutic results? This mystery has haunted ECT practice for decades. In the 1940s and 1950s, the mystery gave rise to a number of speculations about possible psychological reasons why ECT worked. The dominant one was probably the psychoanalytic theory that ECT served as a punishment, thus relieving the beleaguered ego from the internal punishment of the superego (see Chapter Four).

Most psychological theories of ECT's efficacy did not presume that it was necessary to produce a convulsion to produce a therapeutic effect. If, for example, the patient felt better because being shocked in the head with electricity relieved the punishing superego of its duties, it was not clear that the shock also had to cause a convulsion. Nonetheless, early ECT practitioners presumed that the convulsion was a necessary part of the therapeutic process,[82] and this presumption fit their observations, even if no one could say exactly why. The therapeutic need for the convulsion was finally demonstrated by J. O. Ottoson in the early 1960s.[83] Ottoson was a Swedish physician and editor of the important journal *Acta Psychiatrica Scandinavia*, who also produced important work on memory disturbances following ECT and on the use of unilateral ECT.[84] He systematically compared outcomes of patients who received electrical stimulation to the brain with convulsions and without, demonstrating that the convulsion was necessary. From this point on, psychological theories of ECT's efficacy would wither and die; the number of articles on the subject dropped dramatically, and by the 1970s it was not discussed. There was a cost to this, because as inquiry into psychological mechanisms diminished, there was also reduced interest in studying subjective experience of the treatment.

The contrasts between somatic treatments and talk therapies were depicted in many artifacts of popular culture, usually to the disadvantage of somatic treatments. Mary Jane Ward's 1946 novel *The Snake Pit* illustrates this, and is important because of the role it had not only in shaping public views of ECT, but in establishing the asylum novel as a literary form.[85] Widely praised and very popular—it was a Book of the Month Club selection—*The Snake Pit* drew on Ward's experiences during nine months as a psychiatric patient at a New York Hospital.[86] The novel is a story of a woman's descent into a "nervous breakdown," and her experiences in a scary, overcrowded hospital. It appeared at a time of growing public concern about conditions in these hospitals, and its realism was vouched for by some contemporary psychiatrists.[87] In the years after it appeared, de-institutionalization became a nationally enacted policy, one that had many lamentable unanticipated effects, and has received massive criticism from everyone from psychiatrists to radical critics of psychiatry. Yet it is hard to see *Snake Pit* and other documents of mid-twentieth-century mental hospitals without having sympathy for the intentions behind de-institutionalization. The patients are subject to apparent caprices of nurses and doctors in an environment filled with other disturbed people—none of it seems like a place likely to make a suffering person well again. And, with the exception of the devoted emotional work guided by an especially dedicated psychoanalyst, the treatments seem scary.

There is very little depiction of ECT, which is shown alongside older somatic treatments such as hydrotherapy in the book, but ECT was little known to most lay readers when it was released, so the influence of these passages may have been great. Much of the depiction of ECT, consistently referred to as "shock," shows protagonist Virginia Cunningham forgetting about the treatment in between its administrations.[88] This was, to proponents, one of its selling points, as one would not dread what one did not remember. But it is easy to imagine lay readers regarding any treatment that they could forget even having as unsettling. And while there is little suggestion that ECT is used as a punishment, or that it was not therapeutic, the novel does describe the treatments as something you needed to be tied down for, and the patients in the book talk about the therapy as something scary. And, as the novel is an unflattering portrait of the mental hospital overall, ECT had a negative association. The novel, though, does end on a positive note. Virginia recovers, largely through the help of talk therapy with a Dr. Kik, modeled on a psychoanalyst.[89] In the years after the success of the book, though, the coincidentally named Ward continued to face significant challenges from bipolar disorder.[90]

Recall that in her journals, urging herself to make use of her own time in mental hospital as a source of inspiration for a novel, Plath wrote, "I *must* write one about a college girl suicide . . . and a story, a novel even. Must get out SNAKE PIT. There is an increasing market for mental-hospital stuff. I am a fool if I don't relive, recreate it."[91] But the popular 1948 film adaptation starring Olivia de Havilland is more compelling, and more important historically for shaping views of psychiatry and ECT in popular culture. The film probably created a template for future novels and films about asylum life. The film *Snake Pit* even features a cruel and abusive nurse, anticipating the Nurse Ratchet of *Cuckoo's Nest,* and a mute character who reveals she can speak toward the end, like the Chief in *Cuckoo's Nest.* The hospital in *Snake Pit* is depicted as a highly regimented and authoritarian system, where well-meaning doctors and nurses vie with the vindictive ones, who use various forms of discipline, such as transfers to less desirable wards and straitjackets, to punish patients who bother them. Virginia's principal psychiatrist, Dr. Kik, is a stereotypical psychoanalyst, with a pipe and a photo of Freud, who is portrayed very sympathetically. Although his colleagues lack his sensitivity and concern, their deficiencies are also contextualized as the result of the very bad overcrowding in the institution. Kik cures Virginia through classical psychoanalytic means—recovering repressed memories, showing how they relate to repetition compulsions in the present, working through the emotions attached, and evolving from a transference attachment to the analyst. Kik is the hero of the story, whose patient listening and concern for Virginia allow her to avert many disastrous outcomes that are dramatized by chronic cases on the wards.

None of this is possible at the outset, though, because of the psychotic presentation of Virginia at the time of her admission. The ECT is part of a repertoire of shortcuts Kik employs to establish contact with the patient because the crowded hospital requires him to work quickly, although in this regard, the ECT appears to be less effective than the drug-assisted hypnosis, or narcosynthesis Kik employs later. While clinicians at this time were praising ECT for the dramatic reduction in patient fears of convulsive therapy,

Snake Pit dramatizes the fear that remained. Scary movie music plays when the ECT device is shown, and when Virginia sees it she fears she is going to be "electrocuted." But the shock treatments do lead to some improvement in her condition. The film illustrates how a patient helped by ECT might still value psychotherapy for managing their problems. People, whether doctors or patients, rarely concluded in this era that an effective somatic therapy eliminated any need for an understanding of the psychosocial dimensions of a person's life and problems. In his introduction to Ryan and Jessner's textbook, Solomon wondered whether the simple fact of the efficacy of shock treatments meant that psychiatry needed to fundamentally rethink what mental illness was.[92] Such a fundamental rethinking was several decades away, however, awaiting a more favorable cultural moment. In the early years of ECT, both medical and lay culture could view its efficacy as completely compatible with psychoanalytic and other concepts of the self that eschewed biological reductionism.

One thing definitely missing from both the *Snake Pit* book and movie is the relief from symptoms patients experienced and doctors witnessed from ECT. Although ECT is credited as having therapeutic value, mainly as a shortcut that allows the real therapeutic work of psychotherapy to begin, the quick remittance from symptoms is not portrayed. Cunningham's improvement after ECT is shown simply by a notation on her medical chart. We can compare this with the vivid depiction in many clinical reports of the time of patients who had been desperately distressed or despondent for years suddenly having striking recoveries.[93]

"Psychic Driving" and the Costs of Scientific Ambition

> "This paper is concerned with the radical changing of things, with the tearing down and rebuilding of large parts of the understrutting of the world of science in which we work."
>
> Ewen Cameron, 1948[94]

One of the most ambitious attempts to deploy ECT to foster medical progress was also one of the most harmful. This was the experimental therapy called "psychic driving," developed by Ewen Cameron at the Allan Memorial Institute in Montreal.[95] Psychic driving combined large amounts of psychotropic drugs, highly intensive ECT, prolonged sleep, and taped messages, in an attempt to reshape personality. It is a story of an ambitious doctor who did a lot of damage while trying to cure, and also one of nightmares of medical abuse become real.

The idea of progress is not just a descriptor that we can decide to use or withhold as we look at the past. It can also be a powerful mobilizer of the historical actors we study. In the era when medical progress was most ardently believed in, by both the medical and lay communities, the image of the brave and relentless medical researcher taking awesome risks, but bestowing the most priceless of gifts upon humanity, was one that became an ego-ideal for some doctors and scientists. It was an image some sought to bestow on Cerletti, and it was one Cameron sought for himself. While not typical of ECT practice and research, Cameron's work does capture the high hopes and terrible fears of ECT. Cameron provided its history with some of its most ambitious clinical dreams and some of its cruelest results.

Cameron was born in Scotland before immigrating to North America, where he studied with Adolf Meyer. He was an "early adopter" of the new somatic treatments being developed in Europe, was the first to use insulin coma therapy in North America,[96] and argued publicly with colleagues who worried about the dangers of somatic treatments.[97] He was based for most of his career at the Allan Memorial Institute in Montreal. Under his energetic and ambitious leadership, the Allan became a magnet for leading psychiatrists of many subspecialties and for promising psychiatric residents. He also attracted many psychiatric patients who either sought out the best or who were desperate after failed treatments elsewhere.[98]

Psychic driving[99] achieved notoriety, in part because Cameron (possibly without knowing it) received CIA funding. And because it achieved some infamy, it is a story that helps to explain the fear of ECT. His aggressive therapeutic zeal needs to be understood with the recognition that major advances in early twentieth-century psychiatry, such malaria fever therapy, insulin coma, and lobotomy, were invasive treatments, whose risks were considered tolerable only because of the terrible suffering severe mental illness caused. But context is not excuse. I opened this book with the question, hope or horror? Psychic driving may have origins in the search for hope. But its practice and results were clearly horror.

Cameron's approach to psychiatry was not only very aggressive. It was also highly eclectic, drawing on experiments with intensive ECT, new and existing drug treatments, commercial ventures in learning during sleep, sensory isolation practices in intelligence interrogation, and psychoanalysis—the latter a theoretical scaffold he maintained despite his frustration with its slowness in practice. It is striking, in fact, how little interest Cameron's writings show in organic models of mental illness that were often taken up by advocates of somatic treatments at the time.[100] The idea behind the treatment was to use ECT to break down the patient's established personality structure, and then build it up in a healthier fashion through the use of suggestions (first recited live, later taped) read to the patient while the latter was sleeping.

As the CIA pointed out when their funding of Cameron's work was made public, psychic driving was a treatment that he was pursuing anyway. They were not initiating the research, but "buying off the shelf." CIA funding, though, unquestionably helped to sustain and expand the scale of the work, so it's necessary to give some background on the agency's interest. In some ways, it was motivated by the same spirit of "keeping up" with, or ahead of, communist countries that fueled other Cold War scientific projects.[101]

American intelligence officials became convinced that the Soviet Union and China had developed methods of "brainwashing," and wished to follow suit. In a project that came to be called MKUltra, this led to direct research by the CIA itself, as well as funding of academics through a number of front organizations used to foster academic legitimacy. The front organizations included the Society for the Investigation of Human Ecology (SIHE), which also funded research by luminaries including Carl Rogers, Margaret Mead, and B. F. Skinner. Perhaps most incredibly, the list also includes Erving Goffman, whose work on mental hospitals helped to sear in the public imagination the image that they were disciplinary institutions.[102] Some of the CIA research involved dosing uninformed subjects with psychedelic drugs such as mescaline or LSD, sometimes with horrific effects. This was the context in which Hoch and a colleague gave forced injections of mescaline, leading to the death of Harold Blauer.[103] Microbiologist Frank Olson, who was working with the American military, was given LSD without his knowledge, and jumped to his death out of the window of a New York City hotel room.[104] In the midst of these inquiries, the CIA developed an interest in ECT, not because of its therapeutic effects, but because of its known capacity for creating disorientation and memory loss, the possibility that sensitive information could be gleaned from subjects in the stupor following an ECT treatment, and the possibility that it could be used in deliberately painful ways as a form of torture.[105]

With this background, the CIA became aware of Cameron's work on "psychic driving," and decided to finance it. The SIHE approached Cameron, whose work was at that time underfunded despite his energetic efforts to find financial backing. I have seen no evidence that Cameron knew that the CIA was the ultimate source of the SIHE.[106] Anne Collins has suggested he could have figured it out if he had cared to investigate, but on the other hand, the CIA did deliberately try to keep him unaware.[107] Colleagues questioned later had divided opinions on whether Cameron knew.[108] In the context of the early Cold War, many prominent behavioral scientists were not only willing to accept CIA funding, but viewed doing so as part of a patriotic effort. Cameron and the agency had, in any event, compatible agendas. For, just as the CIA was interested in ECT and psychic driving for their possible non-therapeutic applications, Cameron was himself unabashedly interested in brainwashing research, because of what he hoped would be its therapeutic uses.

The ECT Cameron used was a particularly intense form, one that was not the standard of care. Psychiatrists R. J. Russell and L. G. M. Page pioneered intensive ECT in the late 1940s and early 1950s in the United Kingdom.[109] Their therapy was "intensive" in two ways. First of all, it was administered every day; in an aside typical of some defensiveness in a 1953 article they published, they corrected a misperception that it was administered more than once a day. The therapy was also intensive because it increased the electrical stimulus, with the effect of lengthening the tonic phase of the seizure.

This could eliminate the clonic phase, making ECT less dangerous, with reduced risk of bone fracture, and eliminating the need for muscle relaxants. Page and Russell were hopeful that early application of this procedure might prevent new incidences of psychosis from becoming chronic.

Clinicians who used and published about ECT in its first decades—Kalinowsky and Hoch prominent among them—commonly claimed that critics of the treatment were typically people who had no firsthand experience of it, and were therefore motivated by prejudice. Russell and Page adopted the same rhetoric about their variant of the treatment, fending off suspicion apparently held even among ECT providers. For example, they promoted their method as a way to relieve the fear of ECT common in patients, claiming that their patients were no longer afraid after one treatment. They also denied claims that intensive ECT caused more cognitive deficits than normal ECT, saying the deficits were about the same. Yet for Cameron, it was precisely the prospect of creating memory loss that was attractive.

Cameron also took up a psychological fad of the time that was more commercial, sleep learning. The method sought to use the unconscious in learning by playing repeated messages during sleep. For example, nail biters at a summer camp were given a tape that said, "My fingernails taste terribly bitter." Cameron's enthusiasm for sleep learning outlasted that of most other scientists, though.[110]

There are a number of features of Cameron's biography that make his clinical career ironic. His later disgrace—there is even a rock song entitled "The Damning of Ewen Cameron," which has no lyrics, but a dirge-like quality one could call driving—would hardly have been anticipated, given his eminence. He was one of the most celebrated psychiatrists of the mid-twentieth century, and was elected president of several major medical associations. Explanations of why people went along with his methods refer primarily to his distinguished reputation. While his late treatments can be considered prime examples of medical abuse, he was chosen to be among the American physicians consulted in the judgment of medical atrocities of the Holocaust at Nuremberg, atrocities he was very troubled by.[111] If his legacy has been tainted by his association with unsavory intelligence practices of the Cold War era, he was also an outspoken critic of McCarthyism.[112] Further, the man held responsible by many former patients for devastating memory loss had a career-long interest in memory, which he considered (with good reason) to be the foundation of the person.[113] And, while he came to be reviled for causing irreversible damages in his patients, he developed psychic driving in part as an alternative to lobotomy, a contemporary psychiatric practice that Cameron rejected precisely because he feared it would cause irreversible mental deficits.

These ironies can be partly accounted for by his desire for quick treatments. The aggressiveness of psychic driving might be thought of as an attempt to marry the fast action of the new somatic treatments with the long-term reshaping of character thought to be achieved by psychoanalysis.

Cameron combined Russell-Page intensity ECT, at two or more treatments a day, with prolonged sleep therapy induced through the administration of three different barbiturates, antipsychotic medications, and the constant running of audiotapes over 15 to 30 days, although sometimes up to 65 days, intended to suggest changes in the patient's character. The hypothesis behind this regimen was Cameron's belief in "differential amnesia." His hope—and it cannot be described as much more than a hope, because the scientific basis for it was weak—was that patients could lose their schizophrenic memory structures, but regain their normal ones.[114] The ECT was part of a dedicated attempt to break down old patterns of thought and personality.

Note again that this was an attempt to *induce* memory loss. Throughout the history of ECT, memory loss has usually been seen as an adverse effect, with supporters of the treatment tending to see it as rare, and detractors seeing it as common. There have been occasional claims that memory loss is actually the reason for therapeutic effects. The theory is that it erases traumatic or troubling memories. This is not now a widely held view among people familiar with the clinical science.[115] For Cameron, though, memory loss was not only the most valuable part of ECT,[116] but he hoped in fact to deepen it, so that rather than simply losing a few random memories, deeply etched patterns of character could be erased and replaced.

Psychic driving was theorized as a treatment for schizophrenia, and its initial appeal can be understood as a dramatic intervention for very ill people with little hope to be found from other remedies. Nurses explained that they were eager to assist Cameron because he was eager to treat the hopeless cases that other clinicians had given up on.[117] But even in this context it had a shoddy scientific background. The hypotheses on which it was based were poorly developed, and amounted to little more than Cameron's intuition. Given this, it was a cruel treatment even for the very sick. And it was not limited to use on people with chronic psychoses.[118]

One example has been related in detail by the son of a patient. Harvey Weinstein became a psychiatrist himself in part as an attempt to understand what had happened to his father.[119] In addition to his own memories of the course of his father's life and treatment, Harvey Weinstein worked at the Allan as a psychiatrist, where he had access to his father's medical records. Louis Weinstein was a successful Montreal merchant and convivial family man. In 1955, following an examination for kidney stones, he began to suffer from anxiety and panic attacks, and he entered a psychotherapy, which he found unsatisfactory. Seeking the medical care with the best reputation, he then went into treatment with Cameron at the Allan. Cameron's notes on first encountering Louis refer to "anxiety hysteria" and "conversion symptoms."[120] There was no hint of psychosis. Upon entering treatment at the Allan, he complained about the facility, but his complaints were seen as symptomatic of his illness, and only drew the annoyance of the staff.[121] He was given sleep treatment, chlorpromazine, and Russell-Page ECT. After seven ECT treatments "he no longer cared about his business and showed clear memory deficit," and he also lost a tooth.[122] The memory loss immediately following ECT is far from unusual; Russell and Page acknowledged that memory losses were common following their treatment, as it is following mainstream ECT, but they said the memories would generally return, as it often does following mainstream ECT. According to Harvey, though, his father suffered permanent cognitive and affective problems. His anxiety actually was diminished, but he suffered from apathy and depression for the rest of his life, a loss of mental acumen, and permanent memory losses.

Another publicly documented case is that of Val Orlikow, the wife of a Canadian politician, David Orlikow. Val was in a distraught state after the very difficult birth of their child in 1949, two years after they got married.[123] The Orlikows traveled from Winnipeg to the Mayo Clinic, where Val received the vague diagnosis of "character neurosis." Winnipeg at that time had very few psychiatrists, and not a single psychotherapist. She began treatment with a psychiatrist who mainly prescribed Seconal, for sleep, and Val had easy access because her husband had been a pharmacist who owned a drugstore before he entered politics. After four years, she requested ECT, having heard that it provided relief to some, but it did not help. David also procured Largactil (chlorpromazine) for her, before it was generally available, but it had adverse effects. In 1955, she got pregnant again, opted for an abortion, and several doctors agreed that she should have a tubal ligation, a decision none of them told her or David about until she was presented with a consent form for it, which she ultimately signed. Then in 1956, having endured seven years of misery, she learned of the Allan Memorial Institute from her Winnipeg psychiatrist, and she traveled to Montreal.

Val's treatment was a combination of the worst of psychoanalytic assumptions with the most devastating excesses of somatic treatment. Cameron and his team were Freudian enough to interpret her distress as psychogenic, and to interpret any resistance to treatment as a transference-based hostility to authority, rooted in rebellion against her parents. Cameron and some colleagues wrote about Val's case in a research paper, identifying her as "Miriam, a 46-year-old woman who suffers from such intense ambivalence that it has quite destroyed her domestic life."[124] Val's positive transference was illustrated by her comment, "Doctor, you are all things to me," which she said after a period of some psychic driving. This was not uncommon. Cameron seems to have been a charismatic figure, one to whom patients got attached. But after a little more psychic driving she began to show signs of hostility toward the treatment and the nurses, finally telling Cameron, "I don't think I even like you anymore either." The authors did not consider that perhaps this might be due to any problem with the therapy, but saw it more as resistance to the difficult material they were uncovering— but because the case was mentioned so briefly in the paper, there was no discussion of the psychic conflicts involved that would allow us now to make a judgment either way.

But again, Cameron's psychological assumptions were completely Freudian; he just hated the slowness of Freudian therapy. In order to break down her resistance and her personality, he injected LSD—a drug he had little experience with—and amphetamines.[125] She became increasingly resistant to the injections, saying (by her own account), "Okay, I'll do it but I don't want to do it. It's killing me. It's killing me."[126] She came to hide in the bathroom when she heard Cameron coming near on rounds.

Val was discharged, and began to use Cameron's psychic driving tapes on an outpatient basis. On a later re-admission, she was given sodium amytal instead of LSD, and her tapes told her repeatedly that she was "hostile." Cameron then added ECT, but neither he nor Val was optimistic that it would work. Collins writes,

> ECT brought visions of the room they called the sleep room into Val's head. She always kept to the other side of the hall when she had to go by it—people were drugged into sleep for days and days in there and given ECT until they didn't know who they were or where they were or how to feed themselves . . . until they lost control of their bladders and bowels. She saw patients who had just come out of the sleep room standing in puddles of urine in the halls. Banging into walls as they tried to walk. The tapes played there, through speakers under the sleepers' pillows. Val thought people really lost their minds in there. A friend of hers had disappeared after sleep treatment; someone saw her months later, nearly unrecognizable and unable to speak, at the Verdun Protestant Hospital, the place they sent the hopeless cases.[127]

Many other patients had fear of "the sleep room."[128] Ultimately, Val's ability to read was destroyed.[129] The Orlikow family brought suit against the United States government, ultimately winning an award of $750,000 in 1988. The CIA conceded that she had been abused.[130] A *New York Times* article about the settlement mentioned her along with the case of Linda McDonald, a patient of Cameron's who, on discharge, could not remember her husband or children or any of the first 26 years of her life, could not read or write, and had to be toilet trained.

Not surprisingly, especially in retrospect, there is little evidence that the treatment helped any patients, and a number of patients reported very severe memory and cognitive deficits.[131] Given these disturbing stories of permanent memory loss, cognitive decline, incontinence, and other iatrogenic problems, the question of how the practice continued arises. Cameron's charisma, the precedent of other very aggressive somatic treatments, and the lack of good options for severely ill patients did all play a role. It seems likely that those who worked with Cameron were willing to further this aggressive treatment because at least some of the patients were perceived as nearly hopeless cases anyway, but as we have seen, not all of them were. With many abandoned medical treatments, from heroic blood-letting to lobotomy, one can point to perceptions, on the part of clinicians as well as patients and their families, that the treatment worked, even if they seem in retrospect to have either suspect scientific basis or unaccept-able adverse effects. In the case of psychic driving, there is little in the way of even perception of therapeutic success to point to. Published accounts do include the story of Karralynn Schreck, who was diagnosed with "extremely severe anxiety hysteria," and who felt helped by Cameron, expressing last-ing relief and gratitude. But Schreck was admitted in 1962, when full-bore psychic driving was winding down. She was treated with a scaled-down version, with drugs and short sessions with tapes.[132]

After trying psychic driving for nearly a decade, Cameron himself began to suspect its failure. In 1963 he admitted as much to a professional audi-ence in New York.[133] Psychic driving, which already had its doubters at the Allan, was discontinued completely by Robert Cleghorn, Cameron's succes-sor as director of the institute. Cleghorn also reviewed Cameron's work, and found evidence of permanent memory damage to the patients.[134]

Harvey Weinstein's account of psychic driving is remarkably even-handed in its attempt to understand Cameron sympathetically, given Harvey's acknowledged trauma and bitterness over the damage done to his father. But it is not uncritical. Assessing Cameron's motivations, Weinstein sug-gests that Cameron had a "therapeutic zeal that borders on the sadistic."[135] This judgment echoes the views some mid-twentieth-century psychoanalysts had about the spread of a number of somatic treatments, including insulin coma, lobotomy, and convulsive therapy. As I detail in Chapter Four, psy-choanalytic views were varied, but those analysts most opposed to somatic treatments sometimes proposed that the use of these treatments originated in unconscious hostility toward the mentally ill.[136] For a historian, a judg-ment like this could only be speculative. But we do need to ask how to assess Cameron's experiment. Cameron was, at least on the surface, genuinely interested in helping patients and advancing medical science. He allowed himself to abuse the patients, due to a combination of therapeutic zeal, uncontrolled ambition, and shoddy scientific standards.

A recent newspaper article about Cameron asks whether he may have been judged too harshly in retrospect, and cites a psychiatrist now at McGill, Peter Roper, who argues that medicine today is more carefully scru-tinized and patient-friendly than in Cameron's time.[137] It is also true that psychiatrists were using a lot of aggressive and risky somatic treatments in the middle of the twentieth century, and Cameron was certainly not the only one to do so zealously. Cameron was also far from alone at this time in thinking that patients might benefit from being intentionally regressed.[138]

But historical "context" can too easily become "moral shelter," an excul-patory device.[139] Cameron may have been working at a time of aggressive psychiatric treatments, but he did make choices to develop and continue to use perhaps the most aggressive psychiatry treatments of his time, and had opportunity to see the damage they were doing. He was working at a time when ECT alone was considered too aggressive by some in psychiatry, when Russell-Page ECT was seen as too aggressive by some who used ECT, and that is leaving aside all the other aspects of psychic driving. It is important to also consider that plenty of clinicians who worked with Cameron or knew of his work were very uneasy about it.[140] And despite Cameron's high public profile, virtually no one in the psychiatric profession was trying out psychic driving.[141] Cameron's work was more tolerated than celebrated. It was also not in line with evolving scientific standards. Cameron, for example, actively rejected controlled trials during the era they were becoming the gold standard for clinical research, even though they were explicitly recommended to him.[142] For these reasons, psychic driving cannot be easily counted as ethical even within its historical context. Though Cameron does seem to have had a sincere desire to cure the sick, his ambitions viewed patients more as objects and means, more than as subjects or ends.

The experience of psychic driving illustrates the problem with "progress" as a concept of medical history. Historians frequently attack it as simplistic hagiography, and it can be. But it is also an ideal that can have concretely dangerous consequences. This is the reason why the Frankenstein story is so resonant.

Cameron's experiments also show one of the reasons accounts of ECT's past must attend to its more disturbing aspects, whether or not they are representative practices. As virtually any ECT provider will lament, prospective patients are frequently afraid to undergo the treatment. This fear is often regarded as irrational, or at best based on impressions gleaned from sensationalist movies like *One Flew Over the Cuckoo's Nest*. But psychic driving, a fulfillment of people's most dread fantasies of what could happen if they turn their bodies and agency over to medicine, actually did happen. And people knew about it—articles were published on the front page of the *New York Times,* Anne Collins's book about it made the bestseller list, and a story aired on *60 Minutes.*[143]

ECT was a therapy introduced at a time when lay and medical culture were getting used to dramatic results, a culture ripe for recognition of a wondrous treatment. But ECT, while undoubtedly valued by a wide range of clinicians and patients, was not welcomed as the penicillin of psychiatry. There was never a period in which ECT was not discussed among physicians without at least a shade of defensiveness. It failed to consistently radiate the aura of progress so pervasive in the era of its introduction. This failure should not be attributed solely to irrational prejudices and unfair media treatment, even if both of those have been present. Attempts to radiate an image of medical progress for ECT were thwarted in part by real weaknesses in the science and practice of ECT. The basic mechanism of ECT remains mysterious. Given the strength of the data supporting ECT's efficacy in relieving symptoms, the mystery of how it works might have been a minor problem for the therapy. Medical patients are often willing to forgo knowledge of how a treatment works—if they are pretty sure that it does. In the case of ECT, the mystery of how it does what it is supposed to do was compounded by weaker investigation of the extent to which it does things it is not supposed to do—that is, cause adverse effects. I explore this more in Chapter Seven. But even ECT's potential for adverse effects was not the primary reason it remained a hard pill to swallow in its first decades of use. There was widespread suspicion that ECT was used as a disciplinary tool, rather than a medical therapy.

Notes

1   Frank Kimball, "Hope for Tired Minds," *Hygeia* (December 1946) 906–901 & 946; Frank Kimball, "Hope for Tired Minds," *Hygeia* (January 1947) 36–37, 66–69.
2   On McLean, see Alex Beam, *Gracefully Insane: The Rise and Fall of America's Premier Mental Hospital* (New York: PublicAffairs, 2001).
3   See my review of Thomas Szasz, *Coercion as Cure: A Critical History of Psychiatry* (New Brunswick: Transaction Publishers, 2007) in *Bulletin of the History of Medicine* 83, 4 (Winter 2009) 797–798. Szasz, one of psychiatry's most illustrious critics, includes a chapter on ECT, which he denounces as "iatrogenic epilepsy." Szasz's account includes references to a number of well-known patients who say they have been helped by ECT, but he does not even attempt to address the challenge this poses for his argument.
4   Bert Hansen, *Picturing Medical Progress from Pasteur to Polio: A History of Mass Media Images and Popular Attitudes in America* (New Brunswick: Rutgers University Press, 2009).
5   On Miltown, see Andrea Tone, *The Age of Anxiety: America's Turbulent Affair with Tranquillizers* (New York: Basic Books, 2008).
6   Thelma G. Alper, "An Electric Shock Patient Tells His Story," *Journal of Abnormal and Social Psychology* 43 (1944) 201–210.
7   An influential source has been Susan Reverby and David Rosner, "Introduction: Beyond the Great Doctors," in Susan Reverby and David Rosner, eds., *Health Care in America: Essays in Social History* (Philadelphia: Temple University Press, 1979). For a recent reconsideration see Beth Linker, "Resuscitating the Great Doctor," in Thomas Söderqvist, ed., *The History and Poetics of Scientific Biography* (Burlington: Ashgate, 2007).
8   Alfred Freedman, "Lothar Kalinowsky, M.D., 1899–1992," *Comprehensive Psychiatry* 33, 6 (November/December 1992) 357–358.
9   Richard Abrams, "Lothar Kalinowsky, M.D., 1899–1992," *Convulsive Therapy* 8, 3 (1992) 218–220.
10 Freedman, "Lothar Kalinowsky."
11 "Lothar Kalinowsky, A Psychiatrist, 92; Used Electroshocks," *New York Times,* June 30, 1992; Freedman, "Lothar Kalinowsky."
12 Abrams, "Lothar Kalinowsky, M.D., 1899–1992."
13 Abrams, "Lothar Kalinowsky, M.D., 1899–1992." A clinical trial of ECT was conducted in Britain as early as 1939; see G. E. Berrios, "Early Electroconvulsive Therapy in Britain, France and Germany: A Conceptual History," in Hugh Freeman and German E. Berrios, eds., *150 Years of British Psychiatry, Volume II: The Aftermath* (London: The Athlone Press, 1996).
14 See, for example, Lothar Kalinowsky, "Electric-Convulsion Therapy in Schizophrenia," *The Lancet* (December 9, 1939) 1232–1233.

15 Kalinowsky, "Electric-Convulsion Therapy in Schizophrenia," 1233.
16 Claire Hilton, "An Exploration of the Patient's Experience of Electro-convulsive Therapy in Mid-twentieth Century Creative Literature: A Historical Study With Implications for Practice Today," *Journal of Affective Disorders* 97 (2007) 5–12.
17 Zigmond M. Lebensohn, "The History of Electroconvulsive Therapy and Its Place in American Psychiatry: A Personal Memoir," 40, 3 (May/June 1999) 173–181, gives priority to Almansi and Impastato, but his conclusion is based exclusively on Impastato's testimony, which, as I show below, was suspect, although not necessarily wrong.
18 David J. Impastato, "Beginnings of EST in New York Area," Melvin Sabshin Library and Archives. American Psychiatric Association, Washington, D.C. Historical File, Folder 13, "Electro-convulsive Treatment."
19 Melvin Sabshin Library and Archives. American Psychiatric Association, Washington, D.C. Historical File, Folder 13, "Electro-convulsive Treatment."
20 Sydney E. Pulver, "The First Electroconvulsive Treatment Given in the United States," *American Journal of Psychiatry* 117 (1960–61) 845–846. See also Alverno, "The Origins of Electroconvulsive Therapy," 55.
21 Gabor Gazdag, Max Fink, Gabor S. Ungvari, and Edward Shorter, "Laszlo Meduna's Immigration to the United States in 1939," *Journal of ECT* 26, 2 (June 2010) 79–81.
22 Gazdag, Fink, Ungvari, and Shorter, "Laszlo Meduna's Immigration to the United States in 1939," 79.
23 Victor Gonda, "Treatment of Mental Disorders with Electrically Induced Convulsions," *Diseases of the Nervous System* 2, 844 (March 1941) 84–92.
24 Alverno, "The Origins of Electroconvulsive Therapy," 55.
25 Pulver, "The First Electroconvulsive Treatment Given in the United States," 845.
26 Gonda, "Treatment of Mental Disorders with Electrically Induced Convulsions."
27 Gonda, "Treatment of Mental Disorders with Electrically Induced Convulsions," 88.
28 Gonda, "Treatment of Mental Disorders with Electrically Induced Convulsions," 88.
29 Gonda, "Treatment of Mental Disorders with Electrically Induced Convulsions," 87.
30 Clarence Neymann, "Some Thoughts about Shock Therapy," *Archives of Physical Therapy* 24, 660 (November 1943) 660–663. Impastato inferred that Neymann had to have started use later than Impastato himself, solely on the grounds that he would have published sooner on such a timely subject if he could have. Impastato clearly did not have much insight into those of us who write slowly. David J. Impastato, "Beginnings of EST in Chicago Area," Melvin Sabshin Library and Archives. American Psychiatric Association, Washington, D.C. Historical File, Folder 13, "Electro-convulsive Treatment."
31 Neymann, "Some Thoughts about Shock Therapy," 660.
32 Pulver, "The First Electroconvulsive Treatment Given in the United States," 845.
33 Melvin Sabshin Library and Archives. American Psychiatric Association, Washington, D.C. Historical File, Folder 13, "Electro-convulsive Treatment."
34 Melvin Sabshin Library and Archives. American Psychiatric Association, Washington, D.C. Historical File, Folder 13, "Electro-convulsive Treatment." Many of the documents in this folder are memos or letters composed or received by Impastato, who sought in 1969 to determine the when and where of the first American ECT. He was evidently eager to establish his own as the first, and he discounted other possibilities, sometimes on flimsy evidence.

35 Melvin Sabshin Library and Archives. American Psychiatric Association, Washington, D.C. Historical File, Folder 13, "Electro-convulsive Treatment."

36 David J. Impastato, "Beginnings of EST in Boston Area," Melvin Sabshin Library and Archives. American Psychiatric Association, Washington, D.C. Historical File, Folder 13, "Electro-convulsive Treatment."

37 Abraham Myerson, Louis Feldman, and Isadore Green, "Experience with Electric Shock Therapy in Mental Disease," *New England Journal of Medicine* 224 (1941) 1081–1085.

38 See Rasmussen, *On Speed* on Myerson's role in developing amphetamine treatment for depression.

39 Letter from Mollie L. Schoenberg to David J. Impastato, April 29, 1969, Melvin Sabshin Library and Archives. American Psychiatric Association, Washington, D.C. Historical File, Folder 13, "Electro-convulsive Treatment."

40 Myerson, Feldman, and Green, "Experience with Electric Shock Therapy in Mental Disease," 1011. See also Louis Feldman and F. T. Davis, "An Improved Apparatus for Convulsive Therapy," *Archives of Physical Therapy* 22 (February 1941) 89–91, which also touts ECT's favorable side effect and compliance profile compared to chemical convulsive therapy.

41 Myerson, Feldman, and Green, "Experience with Electric Shock Therapy in Mental Disease," 1012.

42 Myerson, Feldman, and Green, "Experience with Electric Shock Therapy in Mental Disease," 1010.

43 Melvin Sabshin Library and Archives. American Psychiatric Association, Washington, D.C. Historical File, Folder 13, "Electro-convulsive Treatment."

44 Lauren H. Smith, Joseph Hughes, and Donald W. Hastings, "First Impressions of Electroshock Treatment," *Pennsylvania Medical Journal* 44 (January 1941) 452–455.

45 Smith, Hughes, and Hastings, "First Impressions of Electroshock Treatment," 452.

46 On Cincinnati, David J. Impastato, "Beginnings of ECT in Cincinnati Area," typescript, Melvin Sabshin Library and Archives. American Psychiatric Association, Washington, D.C. Historical File, Folder 13, "Electro-convulsive Treatment"; on Washington, D.C., Lebensohn, "The History of Electroconvulsive Therapy and Its Place in American Psychiatry: A Personal Memoir."

47 Pulver, "The First Electroconvulsive Treatment Given in the United States," 845; "Letter from Franklin Offner, Professor of Biophysics, Northwestern University, to Walter E. Barton, M.D., February 5, 1969." Melvin Sabshin Library and Archives. American Psychiatric Association, Washington, D.C. Historical File, Folder 13, "Electro-convulsive Treatment."

48 Renato Almansi and David J. Impastato, "Electrically Induced Convulsions in the Treatment of Mental Diseases," *New York State Journal of Medicine* 40, 17 (September 1, 1940) 1315.

49 David J. Impastato, "Beginnings of EST in New York Area," typescript, Melvin Sabshin Library and Archives. American Psychiatric Association, Washington, D.C. Historical File, Folder 13, "Electro-convulsive Treatment."

50 Almansi and Impastato, "Electrically Induced Convulsions in the Treatment of Mental Diseases," 1315.

51 Almansi and Impastato, "Electrically Induced Convulsions in the Treatment of Mental Diseases," 1315–1316.

52 David J. Impastato, "Beginnings of EST in New York Area," typescript, Melvin Sabshin Library and Archives. American Psychiatric Association, Washington, D.C. Historical File, Folder 13, "Electro-convulsive Treatment."

53 Braslow, *Mental Ills and Bodily Cures,* 100.

54 Benjamin Malzberg, "The Outcome of Electric Shock Therapy in the New York Civil State Hospitals," *Psychiatric Quarterly* 17 (1943) 154–163.

55 David Healy, *The Anti-Depressant Era* (Cambridge: Harvard University Press, 1997), 46; Jack Pressman, *Last Resort: Psychosurgery and the Limits of Medicine* (Cambridge: Cambridge University Press, 1998), 10.

56 Braslow, *Mental Ills and Bodily Cures,* 101–104.

57 Lucie Jessner and V. Gerard Ryan, *Shock Treatment in Psychiatry: A Manual* (New York: Grune and Stratton, 1941).

58 Harry Solomon, Introduction to Lucie Jessner and V. Gerard Ryan, *Shock Treatment in Psychiatry: A Manual,* xi.

59 Lothar B. Kalinowsky and Paul H. Hoch, *Shock Treatments and Other Somatic Procedures in Psychiatry* (New York: Grune and Stratton, 1946).

60 Joseph Wortis, "Remembering Paul Hoch," *Biological Psychiatry* 35 (1994) 901–902; Lothar B. Kalinowsky, "In Memoriam, Paul H. Hoch," in Joseph Zubin and Howard F. Hunt, eds., *Comparative Psychopathology: Animal and Human* (New York: Grune & Stratton, 1967). According to Kalinowsky, Hoch had to leave Germany for political reasons—presumably fleeing persecution by the Nazis, although Kalinowsky is not specific.

61 Wortis, "Remembering Paul Hoch."

62 Kalinowsky, "In Memoriam, Paul H. Hoch," 326.

63 H. Brill, "Paul Hoch: Administrator," *Comprehensive Psychiatry* 6, 2 (April 1965) 67–70; F. A. Freyman, "Tribute to Paul Hoch," *Comprehensive Psychiatry* 6, 2 (April 1965) 67–70; Joseph Zubin, "Paul H. Hoch's Contribution to the American Psychopathological Association," *Comprehensive Psychiatry* 6, 2 (April 1965) 74–77; Sidney Malitz, "Paul Hoch, 1902–1964," *American Journal of Psychiatry* 153, 10 (October 1996) 1339.

64 Malitz, "Paul Hoch, 1902–1964."

65 Joseph B. Treaster, "Army Discloses Man Died in Drug Test It Sponsored," *New York Times,* August 13, 1975. The Army claimed it had received consent from the subjects in the experiment, which Blauer's mother and daughter denied. Dr. Sidney Malitz, who later became head of the Institute and who wrote a glowing tribute about Hoch after Hoch's death, conceded that the experiment was probably conducted without the subjects' consent, noting that at the time of the experiments, the prevailing scientific ethos held that it was improper to inform subjects about such tests, because their expectations would then influence the outcome of the study.

66 Abrams, "Lothar Kalinowsky, M.D., 1899–1992."

67 Kalinowsky and Hoch, *Shock Treatments,* 44.

68 Kalinowsky and Hoch, *Shock Treatments,* 5, 101, 103, 106, 129–130. This was a theme Kalinowsky had advanced earlier as well; see, for example, L. Kalinowsky and S. Eugene Barrera, "Electric Convulsion Therapy in Mental Disorders," *Psychiatric Quarterly* 14, 719 (October 1940) 719–730.

69 Kalinowsky and Hoch, *Shock Treatments,* 130.

70 Kalinowsky and Hoch, *Shock Treatments,* 117.

71 Kalinowsky and Hoch, *Shock Treatments,* 131.

72 Kalinowsky and Hoch, *Shock Treatments,* 134.

73 Kalinowsky and Hoch, *Shock Treatments,* 134.

74 Kalinowsky and Hoch, *Shock Treatments,* 142–143.

75 L. Kalinowsky and S. Eugene Barrera, "Electric Convulsion Therapy in Mental Disorders," *Psychiatric Quarterly* 14, 719 (October 1940) 719–730.

76 A. E. Bennett, "Preventing Traumatic Complications in Convulsive Shock Therapy by Curare," *Journal of the American Medical Association* 114 (1940) 322–324; A. E. Bennett, "Curare: A Preventive of Traumatic Complications in Convulsive Shock Therapy," *American Journal of Psychiatry* 97 (1941) 1040–1060.

77 See Hilton, "An Exploration," and Alan Norton, "In My Own Time: Depression," *British Medical Journal* 2 (1979) 429–430.
78 Ryan and Jessner, *Shock Treatment in Psychiatry,* 73.
79 See, for example, Bennett, "Curare: A Preventive of Traumatic Complications," 1040.
80 Malzberg, "The Outcome of Electric Shock Therapy," 156.
81 See Neymann, "Some Thoughts about Shock Therapy," 662; Myerson, "Experience with Electric Shock Therapy," 1012; Gonda, "Treatment of Mental Disorders with Electrically Induced Convulsions," 85; Kalinowsky and Hoch, *Shock Treatments,* 169, 174, & 176; Burns, "The Scientific Origins of Electroconvulsive Therapy: A Conceptual History."
82 See, for example, Kalinowsky and Barrera, "Electric Convulsion Therapy in Mental Disorders," 721.
83 See J. O. Ottoson, "Experimental Studies of the Mode of Action of Electroconvulsive Therapy," *Acta Psychiatrica Neurologica Scandinavia Supplement* 145 (1960) 1–141 and J. O. Ottoson, "Seizure Characteristics and Therapeutic Efficiency in Electroconvulsive Therapy: An Analysis of the Antidepressive Efficiency of Grand Mal and Lidocaine-Modified Seizures," *Journal of Nervous and Mental Diseases* 135 (1962) 239–251. On Ottoson, see Jan Beskow and Tore Hallstrom, "In Honour of Jan-Otto Ottoson," *Acta Psychiatrica Scandinavia* (1991) 399–400. Fink also credits St. Louis researcher George Ulett with the finding that the convulsion was necessary for therapeutic effect; see Max Fink, "What is an Adequate Treatment in Convulsive Therapy?" *Acta Psychiatrica Scandinavia* 84 (1991) 424–427.
84 Ottoson's work on ECT and memory is discussed in Chapter Six.
85 Mary Jane Ward, *The Snake Pit* (Cutchogue, NY: Buccaneer Books, 1983, originally published 1946).
86 *Current Biography 1946* (H. W. Wilson Co., 1946).
87 *Current Biography 1946* (H. W. Wilson Co., 1946).
88 See for example, Ward, *The Snake Pit,* 31, 73.
89 Carmel McCoubrey, "Dr. Gerard Chrzanowski, Innovative Psychoanalyst, Dies at 87," *New York Times,* November 12, 2000.
90 Yael Ksander, "Mary Jane Ward," http://indianapublicmedia.org/momentofindianahistory/mary-jane-ward, accessed June 4, 2012.
91 Alex Beam, *Gracefully Insane: The Rise and Fall of America's Premier Mental Hospital* (New York: PublicAffairs, 2001).
92 Ryan and Jessner, *Shock Treatment in Psychiatry,* xv.
93 See Bennett, "Curare: A Preventive of Traumatic Complications in Convulsive Shock Therapy," 1053–1055 for examples.
94 D. Ewen Cameron, "The Current Transition in the Conception of Science," *Science* New Series, 107, 2787 (May 28, 1948) 553–558.
95 There are several accounts of Cameron's work. John Marks, in *The Search for the Manchurian Candidate: The CIA and Mind Control* (New York: W. W. Norton and Company, 1979), puts his work in the context of the CIA's wider investigations into mind control. See also Anne Collins, *In the Sleep Room: The Story of the CIA Brainwashing Experiments in Canada* (2nd edition, Toronto: Key Porter Books Limited, 1997, originally published 1988); Harvey Weinstein, *A Father, A Son, and the CIA* (Toronto: James Lorimer and Company, 1988); Don Gillmor, *I Swear by Apollo: Dr. Ewen Cameron and the CIA-Brainwashing Experiments* (Montreal: Eden Press, 1987); Gordon Thomas, *Journey into Madness: The True Story of Secret CIA Mind Control and Medical Abuse* (New York: Bantam Book, 1989).
96 Collins, *In the Sleep Room,* 85–92.

97 In 1938, for example, Cameron criticized Oscar Diethelm for raising these concerns. Collins, *In the Sleep Room*, 97–98.

98 Weinstein, *A Father, A Son, and the CIA.*

99 Cameron successively named his treatment "psychic driving," "accelerated psychotherapy," and "automated psychotherapy." Collins, *In the Sleep Room*, 122. In discussions of Cameron's legacy, "psychic driving" is the name that most "stuck," so that is the one I will use.

100 See, for example, D. Ewen Cameron, Leonard Levy, Thomas Ban, and Leonard Rubenstein, "Automation of Psychotherapy," *Comprehensive Psychiatry* 5, 1 (February 1964) 1–14 as an illustration of how deeply saturated in Freudian assumptions Cameron's practice was.

101 See, for example, Audra Wolfe, *Competing with the Soviets: Science, Technology, and the State in Cold War America* (Baltimore: The Johns Hopkins University Press, 2013).

102 Marks, *Search for the Manchurian Candidate*, 168–171. Rogers, for one, was aware that the finds were CIA-sourced.

103 Marks, *Search for the Manchurian Candidate*, 72. Cattell later told Army investigators, "We didn't know if it was dog piss or what it was we were giving him."

104 Collins, *In the Sleep Room*, 29. The United States government admitted culpability during the presidency of Gerald Ford, and Olson's heirs were awarded $750,000 in damages.

105 Marks, *Search for the Manchurian Candidate*, 27–28.

106 Marks, *Search for the Manchurian Candidate*, 98.

107 Collins, *In the Sleep Room*, 137–139.

108 Gillmor, *I Swear by Apollo*, 96–98.

109 R. J. Russell, L. G. M. Page, and R. L. Jillett, "Intensified Electroconvulsant Therapy: Review of Five Years' Experience," *The Lancet* 262, 5 (December 1953) 1177–1179.

110 Gillmor, *I Swear by Apollo*, 46–47.

111 Weinstein, *A Father, A Son, and the CIA*, 90–91.

112 Collins, *In the Sleep Room*, 62–63.

113 Weinstein, *A Father, A Son, and the CIA*, 88.

114 Marks, *The Search for the Manchurian Candidate*, 142.

115 The theory that memory loss was the cause of therapeutic benefits has been criticized on the grounds that no correlation has been found between the extent of memory loss and therapeutic benefit.

116 Collins, *In the Sleep Room*, 130.

117 Collins, *In the Sleep Room*, 165.

118 One example was Mary Morrow, who seems to have been entrapped into the treatment. Weinstein, *A Father, A Son, and the CIA*, 163.

119 My account of the case of Louis Weinstein is drawn from Weinstein, *A Father, A Son, and the CIA*, the book by Louis's son, Harvey.

120 Weinstein, *A Father, A Son, and the CIA*, 34–35.

121 Weinstein, *A Father, A Son, and the CIA*, 36–39.

122 Weinstein, *A Father, A Son, and the CIA*, 43–46.

123 Collins, *In the Sleep Room*, 6–7. Collins applies the term "post-partum depression." The Orlikows were also concerned about Val's loss of interest in sex, although according to Collins's account, Val was mostly concerned about her husband's concern. My account of Val Orlikow is based on *In the Sleep Room*, 6–20.

124 Cameron et al., "Automation of Psychotherapy," 10.

125 On the therapeutic uses of LSD in this period, see Erica Dyck, *Psychedelic Psychiatry: LSD from Clinic to Campus* (Baltimore: The Johns Hopkins University Press, 2008).

126 Collins, *In the Sleep Room*, 15.
127 Collins, *In the Sleep Room*, 20.
128 Marks, *The Search for the Manchurian Candidate*, 143.
129 Clyde Farnsworth, "Canada Will Pay 50's Test Victims," *New York Times*, November 19, 1992.
130 Collins, *In the Sleep Room*, 212–214.
131 Collins, *In the Sleep Room*, 190–196.
132 On Schreck, see Collins, *In the Sleep Room*, 190–196 and Gillmor, *I Swear by Apollo*, 118–119.
133 Collins, *In the Sleep Room*, 188–189.
134 Marks, *The Search for the Manchurian Candidate*, 149.
135 Weinstein, *A Father, A Son, and the CIA*, 41.
136 Prominent analysts who held this view included Otto Fenichel and Gregory Zilboorg. Fenichel was actually in some ways a moderate, in that he thought Harry Stack Sullivan's attacks on somatic treatments were too radical; see Chapter Four.
137 "Stunning Tale of Brainwashing, the CIA and an Unsuspecting Scots Researcher," *The Scotsman*, November 13, 2013, http://www.scotsman.com/news/stunning-tale-of-brainwashing-the-cia-and-an-unsuspecting-scots-researcher-1-466144, accessed November 13, 2013.
138 This is especially clear in Raz's account of Walter Freeman, *The Lobotomy Letters*, ch. 5.
139 The term "moral shelter" developed from conversations I have had with Susan Reverby about the dangers of using "context" as an exculpatory framework for the perpetrators of the notorious Tuskegee syphilis study.
140 Weinstein, *A Father, A Son, and the CIA*, 100.
141 Weinstein, *A Father, A Son, and the CIA*, 104.
142 Gillmor, *I Swear by Apollo*, 92–93.
143 Weinstein, *A Father, A Son, and the CIA*, 84.

3   Therapeutic Disciplines

In the late 1940s, a 23-year-old African-American man in Connecticut received ECT for "homosexuality, transvestism, and psychosis."[1] His doctor, Samuel Liebman, was pleased to have a patient with these combined presentations, because of the opportunity he saw to study their interaction. Homosexuality was widely regarded by physicians as an illness at this time, and ECT was sometimes used to treat it. This does not seem to have been a common use of ECT, which was mainly indicated for schizophrenia and affective disorders, although this is cold comfort to the gay and lesbian people who received ECT, and were traumatized by it.[2]

Liebman described the events leading up to his admission to the hospital:

> He . . . began running around in buses between several of the cities about Hartford 'making a general spectacle of himself.' He went into beauty parlors for permanent waves, walked the floors in department stores as though he belonged there, and when he appeared in court for the evasion of bus fare, he wore curlers in his hair and presented a generally feminine make-up.
>
> In court, the patient said that he had an engagement at eleven o'clock to buy a Packard and get a chauffeur, that he had impersonated females on the stage, and had an appointment to sing in Hollywood that night. He continued stating that he belonged to a nudist camp but refused to stay there because they 'played leap frog.'
>
> On November 15, 1941, the patient was admitted to the Norwich State Hospital.[3]

Shortly after his admission, the patient said:

> I was supposed to be married as one of the Ink-Spots tonight. I'm a woman impersonator. I am going to be married December 24. I will have a white wedding gown with white satin slippers and a long train. It will be a military wedding. I don't want my boyfriend to find out I am here. He is easily excited and might not marry me. We have been going together five years. I am marrying him just for companionship. I have

a half-million dollars and I am going to build three houses—one in California, one in Canada and the other some place in New England.[4]

He was given several ECT treatments over the next few months, after which, his physician reported that he stopped having delusions, and also gave up his cross-dressing. He did not give up his sexual preference, though, and was open and unashamed about it:

> What on earth ever made me act like I did before I came here? No wonder they locked me up, I must have been crazy. . . . I wonder why I acted like that. I know I'm a homosexual. Some of the best people in H. are . . .[5]

This patient clearly did not internalize the view that his sexuality was an illness. But it is also notable that the aspect of his presentation that would continue to be regarded as illness today—his delusions—does seem to have been successfully treated with ECT. This, at least, seems to have been the patient's view, and although his words are given to us through the doctor, it seems unlikely that the doctor would distort this while leaving his rejection of an illness model for homosexuality intact.

The case provides another illustration of the ambiguities in the history of ECT. The treatment provided a clinical benefit for which the patient was grateful. And, from our perspective over a half-century later, the changes following his treatment are not entirely surprising. The delusions, which we would now still consider symptoms of illness, were dispelled. The sexual preference, which medicine has re-evaluated due to successful patient protest, and then discarded as an illness category, was left unaffected.[6] The third "symptom" that interested Liebman, cross-dressing, was dispelled, and while we would not now regard this as a symptom of illness, the patient in this case did.[7] From his point of view, it seems, his illness episode led him to transgress in ways he would not normally.

However medical Liebman's intentions may have been, they need to be considered in the context of overlapping pressures of conformity characteristic of the early Cold War era. If being gay and African-American have been challenging throughout American history, Liebman's patient would have faced the additional challenge at this time of an anti-gay backlash against some liberalization of attitudes that occurred during the New Deal and World War II.[8] This backlash, David K. Johnson has shown, was embedded in the culture of the Cold War, as homophobia was increasingly linked to the fears of communism. If it would be unfair to deny any therapeutic dimension to Liebman's treatment, it is equally hard to see it as a purely therapeutic event.

Psychiatry is a distinctive (although not unique) part of medicine in its reliance on behavior and subjective expression to make diagnoses and warrant treatment. It also can often bring about involuntary treatments, and while that ability may vary, non-legal social pressures to undergo treatment are often present. These two features of psychiatry have often led to the criticism that psychiatry is not so much a branch of medicine as an arm of social control. This line of argument has been taken to the extreme of arguing that mental illness is not really illness at all,[9] although it has more moderate variants. In all of its forms, though, it has usually taken special aim at somatic treatments like convulsive therapies and drugs.[10] This is the background for much of the controversy surrounding ECT. The background can be seen in microcosm in the strong feelings stirred by the film *Cuckoo's Nest,* where a lively non-conformist, who is in no way ill, faces social death by means of somatic psychiatry, an image seared into the consciousness of the American public, to the frustration of those who promote ECT as restorative medicine.

There are critics of ECT use who do not question the reality of mental illness or ECT's ability to relieve symptoms. Still, through much of its history, debate about ECT has hinged upon this basic question: is it in essence a form of therapy as it its name suggests, or does the name mask the reality that it is in essence a technology of social control? The trouble with this way of thinking is that it can be either, depending upon how it is used and in what contexts. But it is also neither, in essence. In its uses and effects, ECT has demonstrably been both—sometimes in the same patient.

This chapter elaborates two major points. First, I want to show in detail how therapy and control are not mutually exclusive goals. This does not mean that they are combined in equal measure at all times. In ECT's early decades, therapeutic and disciplinary aims were combined, sometimes with the therapeutic in the foreground, sometimes the disciplinary. The value of emphasizing this is that it further helps escape the either/or arguments that overwhelm so much debate on ECT's history.

A second major point that emerges from this chapter is that, whatever one's opinion of current ECT use, it is a therapy that has a troubling history, troubles that go beyond the excesses of Ewen Cameron. This matters because fear of ECT is often written off as irrational prejudice or the product of seeing bad movies. While some of the movies may be sensational or misleading, the cinematic trope of the clinician wielding ECT for abusive or controlling purposes is based on the reality that this has happened. ECT proponents may fairly argue "that's not what it's like anymore," but fear of ECT derives not simply from prejudice, but from a social memory of uses that were fearsome. This reality also contributed to the wider critique of psychiatry that would flourish in the 1960s, where coercion to conformity would be figured not as a distortion or side effect of psychiatry's mission, but its core function. As we will see in Chapter Five, ECT would garner particular criticism.

To explore these themes, this chapter develops the concept of "therapeutic discipline," outlined by Braslow in his book on early twentieth-century somatic treatments. Focusing on Stockton State Hospital in California,

Braslow showed that for several treatments, including hydrotherapy, shock therapies, and lobotomy, managing or controlling patients often combined with therapeutic aims in complex ways, and were often closely allied aims. Specific diagnoses were not, in this hospital, the main predictor of who received ECT, and shock schedules were tailored to the degree of difficulty patients showed. Highly agitated patients received a "blitz" method, with shock treatments every four hours.[11] Braslow stresses that these practices stemmed from the premises of therapeutic discipline. From the clinicians' point of view, getting the patients under control was of a piece with making them better, as their unruliness was seen as a symptom.

Recognizing the kinship—sometimes close, sometimes more distant—between control and therapy does not mean denying political or moral distinctions about how a therapy has been used. It is possible to identify troubling degrees of coerciveness in ECT practices, or any psychiatric or psychological practices, without concluding such ends were purely coercive. Similarly, it is possible to find instances where therapeutic goals seem to have been predominant, and where that aim tallied with patients' subjective assessment, and still recognize that controlling undesired behavior was an element of the process. The concept of therapeutic discipline allows us to place particular uses of a treatment along a spectrum, rather than insisting that the treatment is in its essence purely coercive, or purely therapeutic.

Historians of psychiatry have gotten into many heated, and some would say interminable, debates over whether psychiatry should be seen as "social control."[12] People who are not in the field may in fact find it hard to believe how much debate there has been over whether the history of psychiatry should be seen as a history of therapy or as a history of coercion.[13] These debates have been far from fruitless; they have stimulated good research, and sharpened debate over the role of psychiatry in society. Some—a small minority of people who have participated in these discussions, really—have taken the extreme view that psychiatry is *only* social control, in a most malevolent sense.[14] While this extreme view may not be widely persuasive, it has helped to illuminate darker reaches of psychiatric practice, and to foreground the elements of social control at work even when psychiatry is at its most therapeutic and benign.

There are at least two good reasons why these debates have been so heated, and so repetitive. One is that they touch on a basic tension inherent in the practice of psychiatry. The other is that the term "social control" itself has had shifting usages, and these differing usages have very different moral valences. It is common for this kind of malleability of meaning of key terms to afflict scholarly debates. Another example, closely related to but definitely distinct from "social control," is the vast literature on "social construction" that flourished especially in the 1990s, being applied to virtually everything.[15] The term was controversial in the many domains of nature and society to which it was applied, but its application to psychiatric categories sparked some very vivid discussion. The nub of the problem, often, was that scholars of a more positivist bent often took the "social constructionists" to be saying that mental illness was not "real," although things that are created by society—race, class, gender, the tax code—are very real, and being real does not mean preceding human agency.

In other words, people are not always talking about the same thing. In the case of social control, the term can, for example, be used to refer to the blatantly abusive practices of Soviet psychiatry, where the trappings of medicine were used cynically for purposes of deliberate political oppression. To a critic of psychiatry like Thomas Szasz, that is only marginally different—if at all—from what psychiatry is always doing. That is, if mental illness is a myth, and psychiatry not properly a branch of medicine, then the only thing separating Soviet psychiatry from any other is some light shading of cynicism in intent. But the term "social control" can also be used in a more descriptive, less denunciatory, sense. The sociologist Allen Horwitz, who has written extensively on psychiatry and social control, points out that the term social control had a very wide meaning when it was introduced into American social science in the early twentieth century, referring to any of the many ways society works to re-establish normative order, and not limited to coercive or punitive ways.[16]

Medicine, of all kinds, always operates to return people to their social roles. This is most obvious for psychiatry, because for the most part psychiatric symptoms, whether believed to be caused by biology or life events, are assessed by measuring deviance from social norms; there are no blood tests or visible lesions for psychiatric diagnoses. But the treatments of malaria, influenza, cancer, and broken bones also attempt to return the individual to their social roles. This is one of the key insights of Talcott Parsons's medical sociology. To Parsons the "sick role" was an example of deviance from normal social roles, but deviance that was sanctioned.[17] A sick person was, in this model, allowed to stop making normal contributions to society in terms of work productivity, for example. But this sanctioning of deviance had limits, according to Parsons. Adopting the social role also meant adopting certain social obligations. Above all, the person occupying the sick role is obliged to try to get better, and to submit to the authority of medical experts by doing what they say the sick person should do to get better. Parsons's theory was influential, and has also had its critics. Its use has declined in sociology, according to John Burnham, because of changing intellectual priorities within that discipline.[18] I also think that, with its emphasis on the obligation of the sick person to comply with medical advice to get well, it was perfectly suited for an optimistic moment in medical history when cures for infectious diseases were becoming more common and the intractability of chronic conditions not as glaringly obvious as they would come to be. Yet with its limitations, Parsons's conception contained a durable insight: that being sick can mean a departure from one's usual social expectations, and medicine's role—in addition to its other roles, such as reducing pain and suffering and prolonging life—is to return people to their previous roles. Often, this is exactly what people want from medicine.

ECT was introduced into American society during World War II, and it became a major part of psychiatry's therapeutic repertoire during the early years of the Cold War. Americans remember this period with both nostalgia and distaste, as a time of powerful pressures to conformity. There is, of course, some merit to this historical memory. These were years when, for example, McCarthyism created intense incentives to avoid even the appearance of radical political dissent, years when suburban domestic ideals about the nuclear family made gender roles rigid. As with all historical periodization, we have to be careful to not reduce the era to stereotypes. The 1950s were years of important challenges to the political status quo, such as the Civil Rights movement and important stirrings of the feminist movement. In the realm of culture, while many intellectuals warned about the Man in the Gray Flannel Suit, beatniks were rousing the beginnings of a counter-cultural movement that would flourish in the 1960s, leading also to challenges to psychiatry.

The remainder of this chapter will pursue the ambiguities of therapeutic discipline of ECT in its early decades. It will consider the problem under three main rubrics that have frequently been cited as evidence that ECT has been used as a mechanism of social control: 1) ECT as a tool for maintaining order and hierarchy on the wards of mental hospitals, 2) ECT as a tool for gender conformity, and 3) ECT as a tool for the enforcement of sexual norms.

When looking at medicine as a tool for enforcing social discipline, one cannot, in my view, avoid looking at evidence of illness and treatment. This would be treated as self-evident in the history of, say, infectious disease. But because the study of the etiology of many mental illnesses has not yielded empirical specificity that can rival the methods of Koch's postulates, the field has been open for critics to question diagnostic categories and even whether the model of illness itself is apt. This line of criticism has its own history, one I explore in Chapter Five. I am unpersuaded that mental illness is not in fact illness because it lacks for visible pathogens or lesions. (Why should these be the criteria?) What societies place in the realm of illness and medicine is historically shifting, philosophically complex, and certainly an important area for study. Whether to call a condition or set of symptoms an illness is a social decision, carries in many cases both benefits and disadvantages, and is subject to change.[19] There are obvious cases, such as homosexuality, which went from not an illness, to an illness, and back to not an illness, all over the course of the twentieth century.[20] Another is alcoholism.[21] Perhaps more unexpectedly for some, hearing voices, long medicalized under the rubric of psychosis, is now the subject of a movement among some voice hearers to demedicalize.[22] Many people who hear voices may find this liberating, although some may not. It is worth reflecting, though, that some core symptoms, such as morbid delusions, suicidality, and severe melancholy in the absence of severe cause for grief, have a long history of being considered under medicine's purview, both in Western history and cross-culturally. This does not prove that they are objectively illnesses, but it is reason to reflect on the power the illness model has had.

This model has had power for psychiatric patients, not just the people around them. And while engaging in retrospective diagnosis is problematic, one does not have to fit someone into a diagnostic category to attend to the manifestation of their sickness. The history of psychiatry has ably progressed to where we rightly raise political questions about the diagnoses and treatments of patients. This is an important part of including patients' perspectives. But to err on the opposite extreme, to assume no psychiatric patients were sick in any meaningful way, omits a "patient's perspective," as well. It also transforms the psychiatrists, in effect, into merely sadistic policemen of the social order. This is an impoverished historiography, and one that does a great disservice to people whose suffering has been eased by psychiatry.

ECT and Order on the Wards

ECT providers and others who value ECT bitterly resent the effect of *One Flew Over the Cuckoo's Nest*—the novel, and even more the film. It is possible that there is no other cultural production that so ominously dominates the public consciousness of a medical treatment. *Cuckoo's Nest* portrays ECT—unmodified, that is without anesthesia or muscle relaxants—as a form of control, a way of disciplining patients who do not comply with staff. This depiction does not adequately depict the whole of institutional ECT practice in the 1940s and 1950s, but neither was it merely a product of the imaginations of Ken Kesey, or Milos Forman, who made the film adaptation.

In this section, I cull the evidence from a variety of primary and secondary sources to explore the pull between therapy and control in mental hospitals during the early years of ECT. As we look at various cases, keep in mind that although the muscle relaxants and anesthesia were introduced early, they were not spread uniformly. So even if ECT was used without any punitive intent, it could be a frightening experience. In 1982, the psychologist Norman Endler published a memoir, *Holiday of Darkness,* about his own struggle with depression, and his recovery through ECT.[23] This was an important book in ECT history, because it was one of the first of a number of relatively positive personal accounts that were published starting in the 1980s. Endler's story was not just of a struggle with depression, but with his own decision, as a mental health professional turned patient, to have ECT. His memoir is a conversion narrative. While the decision to get ECT is rarely easy for anyone, Endler was deeply opposed to ECT. His opposition was based on revulsion born from his clinical training, and not based on sensational images in movies.

> My first contact with ECT will provide the 'flavor' of the general atmosphere surrounding it and will also help to explain why I had such a strong negative attitude toward it. During the mid-to-late 1950s I was a graduate student in clinical psychology at the University of Illinois.

As part of our training we were required to study various clinical techniques and procedures, which included ECT. We visited a psychiatric
state hospital on central Illinois to observe patients of various diagnostic categories and how ECT was administered. . . . As I write this, I still
shudder at the memory and still feel the sickness in my stomach. . . . The
patient then was wheeled into the room in his bed, lying on his back.
We were in an observation room a few yards away . . .[24]

No anesthesia was used, the patient was pinned down, and there were violent convulsions and a "blood-curdling yell." Endler believed the patient's
back was broken. There is no indication in Endler's account that the
patient was being intentionally disciplined for an infraction or even any
non-conformity. His teachers had no inhibition showing this spectacle of
unmodified ECT as part of Endler's therapeutic training, because it shows
there was still much progress to be made in establishing modified ECT as
the standard of care.

We do know, though, that ECT in these years was used for blatantly punitive and coercive purposes. The most notorious example is Milledgeville, a
large mental hospital in the Georgia city of the same name. Milledgeville's
infamy was partly incurred because a doctor who worked there, Peter Cranford, wrote an account.[25] Cranford described the hospital's punitive use of
ECT, publicizing what was known there as the "Georgia Power Cocktail."[26]
This usage was at least partly a way of managing a clinical staff shortage
at a time of great overcrowding. By 1942, the hospital had a medical staff
of 15 people for a patient population of 10,000, and so the doctors had
patient loads numbering between 600 and 1,000.[27] Cranford said that "this
produced an unhealthy situation."[28]

The matter of who was to receive electric shock treatment on the various wards was largely based on the reports of nurses and attendants.
The words 'punish' and 'shock treatment' were often synonymous to
the disturbed. Which electric shocks were given for treatment, which
for punishment, and which for both presented confusing problems to
patients, many of whom were paranoid to begin with and felt they were
being punished for their 'guilty' deeds prior to their illness. . . . The
attendant himself was confused when he was criticized for using force
to subdue a patient who might have attacked him when he had heard a
physician say that force was unnecessary 'because shock treatment left
no marks.' The physician could have added that the patient would not
even be able to remember the circumstances surrounding the behavior
leading to the punitive shock treatment.[29]

Cranford's account is critical, but he also acknowledges a therapeutic side of
ECT practice, even at Milledgeville, noting that it was safer and easier than
the chemical treatments that had preceded it, and that with its advent, the
institution had for the first time the appearance of a hospital, the "ravings of

the maniacal completely stilled by the shocking machines."[30] The costs were obviously too high. The abusiveness of these practices is not controversial. The question it raises for the wider history of ECT is, how common was this sort of practice?[31] It is possible that Milledgeville was the worst institution in the United States, and its wards for black inmates were especially horrific.[32] But Milledgeville was far from alone in using ECT for punitive purposes.

One account from this period, Ivan Belknap's *Human Problems in a State Mental Hospital,* mentions that ECT was in the repertoire of rewards and punishments (as a punishment) for uncooperative patients, and in fact had a major role in enforcing order on the wards.[33] When the daily ECT list was made, it would consist of those who were causing trouble, or had become disturbed or violent, plus a number requiring maintenance therapy—which were those with a history of violence, who might get a shock sequence of up to three months. "The amnesia and disorientation produced in these patients by the shock treatment keeps them quiet and prevents their disturbing or hurting the other patients and upsetting the ward routine."[34] Shock lists always included insubordinate patients, and the probability of punitive ECT was greater for patients with lower social status. Attendants named the difficult patients, because the physicians spent so little time on the wards. ECT was, then, structurally separated from its medical purpose. Patients could, according to Belknap, be put on the list because they responded "with normal resentment" toward mistreatment by an attendant or another patient, or for refusing to eat hospital food. He added:

> The sixth level hallucinatory and delusional 'worry warts' were particularly likely to be put on the shock lists. One senior attendant said frankly that he put one of these patients on the list to give himself and the ward a rest from a particularly boring story.[35]

For most patients, the prospect of ECT quickly brought about their compliant behavior. The source of their fear, Belknap said, could not have been their memory of the procedure, because amnesia of the treatment was complete. Rather, there was talk around the hospital about the experience of ECT. Also, patients assisted in the administration, and the procedure was done in plain view.[36] It would have been a spectacle:

> The patient's convulsions often resemble those of an accident victim in death agony and are accompanied by choking gasps and at times by a foaming overflow of saliva from the mouth. . . . Moreover, in the early disorientation and vacuity of his state of recovery he is obviously upsetting to the other patients.[37]

Most patients, and attendants, in the hospital Belknap studied believed ECT was genuinely therapeutic, but there were rumors about broken backs, fatal heart attacks, and brain injury, as well as stories of older patients who died from the strain, and chronic patients whose faculties disintegrated after many treatments. Belknap did not verify whether any of these stories were true, but none of them are implausible. Belknap emphasized that the hospital staff did not explain the procedure to patients, thus leaving fertile ground for rumor.[38]

This hospital replicated a finding that Braslow emphasized in his study of Stockton, namely that the therapy and control of patients were seen by hospital staff as complementary, not as inconsistent objectives.[39] Staff saw ECT as the most effective treatment the hospital had to offer and believed it would promote both physical and mental health. They also genuinely saw disorderly and uncompliant behavior as signs of illness.[40]

At St. Elizabeth's Hospital in Washington, D.C., medical staff used ECT regularly but cautiously, as they had doubts about the claims to safety made by proponents.[41] The primary indications were depression and agitation. This was a case where very conscious efforts were made to keep the focus of ECT on its medical application. Many of the patients, particularly those who were depressed, were amazed at how much better they felt after the ECT.[42] But here too, clinicians deliberately applied ECT to agitated patients as a means of control, admitting that they held out little hope for therapeutic value—in contrast to the higher hopes for ECT in cases of depression. The agitated patients, not surprisingly, tended to be more negative about the treatment.

That physicians and attendants used ECT for disciplinary purposes in mental hospital wards is disturbing. But it is unfortunately not surprising if one is familiar with the history of psychiatry. One does not have to adopt the more conspiratorial views of the field to recognize that. And mental hospitals in the middle of the twentieth century posed special challenges. People with severe mental illnesses can be hard for anyone to deal with in any time and place. Putting them all together in institutions may or may not be a good idea, but even if it is, the most salient fact about the mental hospitals in the mid-twentieth century was their overcrowding, and consequent understaffing. This is why some contemporary accounts claimed that the *primary* goal of the attendants in mental hospitals was to enforce control over the patients.[43] As Goffman pointed out in his classic study of asylums, some antagonism was structured into stereotypical views staff and patients held toward one another, where staff tend to see inmates as "bitter, secretive, and untrustworthy" and inmates tend to see staff as "condescending, highhanded, and mean."[44] He also mentioned that the hospitals sometimes extracted "the teeth of biters, gave hysterectomies to promiscuous female patients, and lobotomies on chronic fighters."[45] The temptation to use a feared treatment, and one that usually left no physical lesions, or memory of the experience, must have been great. Mary Jane Ward's *Snake Pit* became famous for dramatizing fearful aspects of the mental hospital, even though in the end it was a story of successful recovery. Ward went on to agitate for reform of the mental hospitals. She emphasized that even in the better hospitals, patients lived in constant fear of reprisals by staff.[46] Another contemporary account, by John Maurice Grimes, referred to the frequent use of socks filled with bars of soap by attendants, in order to hit patients without leaving marks.[47]

We of course do not have studies documenting ECT use in every hospital in the country. The evidence that we do have says that ECT use in mental hospitals in its first decades was characterized by a spectrum, ranging from the most punitive to the most caring. At the notoriously disciplinary Milledgeville, there was evidence that ECT had therapeutic benefits. And at a famously benign institution like McLean, where there is little evidence of abuse by attendants, the prospect of ECT could be terrifying to patients, at the least.[48] Milledgeville may have had an especially bad reputation, but the attention Milledgeville has received is due to its size, not to its uniquely sinister practices.

In the 1950s, social and intellectual movements condemning psychiatry, and in particular institutionalized psychiatry, and also in particular somatic treatments like ECT, began to simmer, before coming to a full boil in the 1960s. It is not surprising that these movements would seek to recast an arm of medicine as a form of discipline for non-conformists. All too frequently, it was.

What is also striking about this picture is its resemblance to the depiction of ECT in *One Flew Over the Cuckoo's Nest.* Whatever faults there were to *Cuckoo's Nest,* there was nothing that happened in it with regard to ECT that could not have happened in a 1950s mental hospital. The remote physicians, vengeful staff, and especially the punitive use of ECT were all completely plausible. Kesey had worked in a state mental hospital, and had the opportunity to observe these practices.

"Able to Manage Her Home Effectively"

Some of the creative literature of this period would form the foundation of a feminist critique of psychiatry, a critique that would later take a more systematic form in books like Phyllis Chesler's *Women and Madness.* Plath's work is a case in point. Esther Greenwood's path to psychiatric treatment is a response to the contradictory pressures facing an ambitious woman in an era of gender backlash. Plath's representation of ECT, I argued at the outset, is a little more complicated than is often remembered. But it is also by no means one of a straightforward cure—or a straightforward illness.

Were challenges to women's traditional roles "silenced at the push of a button" on an ECT machine, as one account has bluntly put it?[49] There is certainly precedent in the history of psychiatry for its use in muffling voices of protest. And gender occupies a special place in the debates over ECT's role as therapy and control, because women seem to have predominated as ECT patients.[50] There is surely a gender politics to this, but the meaning of the politics cannot be inferred simply by the numbers, because the numbers raise perennially challenging questions of historical epidemiology: were women getting certain illnesses at higher rates than men? If so, what was the source of the gender ratio? Were they getting them at similar rates, but getting diagnosed and treated more? Were diagnosis and treatment rates similar, but ECT used more readily on women with the same diagnosis as the men? It is doubtful that we will be able to answer these questions with certainty based on historical evidence.[51] For one thing, we would need to know a lot about those who went untreated. What we can do is look closely at patient and clinician representations of the path to treatment and the treatment itself with an eye to clues about the role gender played. When we do, we find again that therapy and discipline intermingled in complex ways. The gendering of ECT does not yield a simple story of the silencing of women's complaints, nor of remedying suffering. Braslow's work on Stockton actually included a close look at a case where a woman was supported by her ECT doctors in her quest for independence from her husband.[52] As with the general question of therapeutic discipline in the hospitals, ECT was used for a complex array of reasons for both sexes. Relieving symptoms often blurred with the goal of returning the patient to her social role. And again, these were often seen as the same thing—by both clinician and patient.

There are certainly examples of sexist uses of ECT. For example, Kneeland and Warren cite the example of a book on marriage by an author named Paul Popenoe from 1950 that recommended the use of ECT to handle mood changes associated with the menstrual cycle.[53] I have not seen evidence that this use of ECT was common. On the other hand, Popenoe does mention it casually, as if were unremarkable, suggesting that it might have been common.

This section will look closely at a number of sources from the 1940s and 1950s that have been used to illustrate use of ECT to enforce of gender norms. Many of these sources were not written primarily about gender. There is of course nothing wrong with using sources that were written for other purposes to unearth assumptions about gender. They may, in fact, be all the more revealing about gender if they are not written to be. But it is also important to consider the whole context of the treatment as presented in the sources. There is a substantive difference between giving a person a medical treatment *simply* because she has a complaint about her traditional role, and treating her in the midst of considerable and multifaceted distress that may include some protest against her traditional role.

One source that has been offered as evidence, for example, was a large study of causes of failure in ECT treatment, published in 1947, cited as evidence that the goal of ECT was the conformist one of making women "able to manage her home effectively" and "active in society."[54] One of the authors, N.K. Rickles, had earlier conducted a study of 200 ECT patients in a private Seattle sanitarium, and found an 81% recovery rate. Rickles attributed the high rate of recovery not simply to the ECT, but to follow-up with psychotherapy, and when possible intervention into social conditions that were agitating the condition of the patient. With colleague Charles Polan, he conducted a follow-up analysis of 38 cases where there was no improvement, and found the common factors to include

> history of insidious onset, gradual withdrawal, disharmony of affect, a feeling of being different and inability to feel deeply or to express oneself easily or freely. The presence of conflict over early sexual acts, such as masturbation, homosexual practices, or abortion, was always of poor prognostic significance in these schizophrenic illnesses.[55]

A couple of things stand out in this passage. One is that shame or conflict over socially stigmatized sexual or reproductive choices was not helped by ECT. This is hardly surprising. Their article detailed case studies of patients, both men and women, with severe depression, disorientation, anxiety, suicidality, and other symptoms who, they lamented, had failed to improve, as well as some cases, also of both sexes, who did. In all cases, the ability to leave the hospital well and able to return to something like the life they lived before the onset of illness was the main criteria of success. They were circumspect in admitting the lack of statistical strength to their sample, but were hoping that further research would help to determine with more precision when ECT should be used—and when not. Reducing the article to evidence that ECT was used to enforce the social role of housewife is selective.

Another source used to support the claim that complaints about women's social roles were silenced by ECT is a rich and detailed account of one physician's approach to treating psychosis in the Forest Sanitarium in Des Plaines, Illinois.[56] Julius Steinfeld was a psychoanalytically oriented psychiatrist who used ECT, as many analysts did, in order to provide enough relief of severe symptoms so that insight-oriented analytic work could proceed. As I show in the following chapter, the idea that psychoanalysts were uniformly hostile to somatic treatments is a stereotype read back from our current age of biopsychiatry, not an accurate reflection of the range of psychoanalytic views. Steinfeld wanted to see if dynamic therapy could be used successfully in severely disturbed patients, as opposed to the more modestly neurotic often held to be the more likely candidates. He looked into whether this could be accomplished by using ECT and insulin first. He actually stressed that with the patient population he was treating, dynamic approaches alone would be counter-productive. As was the case with Rickles and Polan's study, Steinfeld's study looked at both male and female patients.[57] And here again therapeutic success was generally measured by the patients' ability to reassume their pre-morbid social role. For many of the women that may have indeed been their role as housewives, but it must be added that when the woman in question was, for example, pursuing a master's degree, therapeutic success was measured by her return to school.[58]

Patients were often relieved to be returned to their ability to fulfill their social role, whatever our view of their social role might now be. There was, for example, a woman described in a 1947 newspaper report who had been homebound and disheveled, frequently weeping, and requiring constant supervision. After six treatments of ECT she resumed management of her household, as well as her leadership in civic organizations. Perhaps even more significantly, she became a virtual ECT evangelist, actively seeking out other people whom she thought would benefit from the treatment.[59]

None of these examples are meant to show that Betty Friedan's famous "problem with no name" was not actually a problem. They are meant, rather, to show that it is a mistake to reduce ECT practice to a quick social fix to silence the problem. Both sides of this point can be illustrated by an illness memoir of the period, Judith Kruger's *My Fight for Sanity* (1959).[60]

Kruger opens her story with the memory of wishing to have a perfect 1950s home and her tremendous desire to have children—the children, in her mind, being largely a gift of repayment to her own parents.[61] She did, though, have some anxieties about parenting, which she managed in classic 1950s fashion—by reading Dr. Spock.[62] After her child was born, a bout of anxiety hurtled rapidly into a breakdown, leading to suicidality and hospitalization. The narrative is not detailed about the period of postpartum struggle until the point where Kruger was in the hospital. Possibly, she did not remember the days before the hospitalization, whether because of the illness or the ECT she received, although she did vividly remember her mounting fear as the time for the ECT drew near. Following her first ECT, she lay down on the ward, learned that she was only gone 40 minutes, and remembered thinking:

> Forty minutes. A short eternity. What is it they do to strip a mind so fast? Electric shock. A shock with electricity. Why? To make me better? Don't feel better. Just so tired. Exhausted. Every muscle . . . every nerve . . . my legs . . . and arms . . . and eyes . . . so tired . . .[63]

The "why?" in this passage matters. It is easy to forget how difficult it can be for patients, no matter how sick they feel themselves to be, to subject themselves to an intense procedure whose rationale is unclear. One may not know how aspirin works, but on the other hand, taking it is no big deal. Nevertheless, Kruger expressed her relief eloquently:

> I woke up . . . at six-thirty. For the first time in eight weeks I had slept. For ten hours. Without sedation. And there was peace. And calm. And a quiet inside me.[64]

Here is the enormous relief of the mentally distressed at relief of symptoms. But Kruger was not a straightforward enthusiast for ECT. In fact, she said she "hated" it, and although her fear of it subsided and she continually noted its therapeutic effects, the rest of the memoir describes avoiding it as much as possible. She also resented the silence of her doctor—"Would it have killed him to say a word of comfort?"[65] Historians of medicine have shown that the development of medical technology can have the effect of increasing personal distance between patient and physician, and this may be most pronounced for psychiatric patients.[66] Upon release from the hospital she underwent a therapy she preferred—talk therapy with an attentive psychoanalyst, whom she valued for his unwillingness to paper over her darker impulses.[67] Also home from the hospital she thought about how little she wanted to be a mother, how drab and demeaning housework was, how much she wanted freedom.[68] One possible reading of Kruger's story is that her psychiatric treatment, rather than silencing her protest, actually allowed her to realize how unhappy she was with her assigned gender role.

Kruger's story also underscores why we cannot avoid questions of efficacy when writing historically about treatments. Kruger was no simple ECT enthusiast. She was, though, clear about the help it gave her. In her words: "Depression depresses. Relief relieves. And the ego springs back. Simple as that. But only when you're out of it."[69] Listening carefully to patients' voices means hearing both the gratitude and the protest, sometimes in the same patient.

"$62,000 for Nothing! You Haven't Changed a Bit"

Few people would regard the use of any medical treatment to return people to their social roles as a bad thing in all instances. This is often the deliberate wish of people who are sick. But we know well by now that the meaning of being "sick" can vary, and the history of psychiatry provides an unusually rich field of changing and debatable illness categories. It also provides, in its changing orientation toward homosexuality, an example of an illness category that was successfully challenged by patients.[70] Prior to that challenge, convulsive therapy was part of the accepted repertoire of treatments.

The development of convulsive therapy coincided with a period of significant backlash against open homosexuality, as well as a period where gay identity would increasingly be tied to sexuality rather than gender identity.[71] It was also a time when living a double life could be a significant source of stress for gay people, whether or not they internalized the social stigma. It was also the era of the "lavender scare," where gay people's persecution was compounded by McCarthyism and they were regarded as a security risk.[72] This, with the medicalization of homosexuality, forms the backdrop to the attempts to use convulsive therapy to alter sexuality—as well as an especially powerful reminder that, as Jennifer Terry has pointed out, medicalization held some promise for gay people, but had dangers as well, and was certainly no insulation against stigma.[73]

Almost all the evidence we have suggests it did not work. That is, there is almost no record of convulsive therapy appearing to alter anyone's sexuality. The one exception is the earliest publication on the question, which not surprisingly used Metrazol. This was a 1940 article by a physician named Newdigate Owensby. Owensby was a psychoanalytically informed doctor who proposed that homosexuality was an "underdeveloped" form of schizophrenia, arrested at the phase of psychosexual development where the libido became fixated, and that the Metrazol would liberate the fixation.[74] Admitting in the title of the piece that it was a "preliminary" study, Owensby treated only six patients, five of them male. He reported success—that is, a change to heterosexuality—in all of the cases. Given that no subsequent attempts at using ECT to alter sexual preference reported success, there are grounds to be skeptical of Owensby's findings. In fact, given how unpleasant we know Metrazol treatment to be, it is plausible that the patients reported changed sexuality in order to avoid any further treatments, but this is speculative.

The small number of other clinical accounts report uniformly "negative" results. One was Liebman's, as we saw at the beginning of this chapter. Another was by George N. Thompson, who provided a report on five patients from Camarillo State Hospital in California where patients had been committed between 1941 and 1942 under the "sexual psychopath law."[75] The law prevented those committed after alleged homosexual crimes from having the prospect of parole unless they were treated and cured. These cases were varied. One was accused of rape, but for most of them their main crime seems to have been simply engaging in homosexual acts. All received either Metrazol or ECT. What is striking is a similarity with Liebman's account: in cases where there were sources of distress less controversially regarded as psychiatric symptoms, such as delusions and hallucinations, there was evidence of symptom remission after the convulsive therapy, and Thompson reported some relief about this from the patients. In no case, however, was there any report of any change of sexual orientation. Thompson concluded that convulsive therapy was of no use for that purpose.

There are a few available accounts of the use of ECT to alter sexuality that provide perspectives of those who underwent the treatment. Jonathan Ned Katz provided an interview with one such case in his documentary history of gays and lesbians in America.[76] This was the case of an anonymous young man, involuntarily committed by his parents to a private mental hospital in the South in the early 1960s at the age of 24 in order to cure his homosexuality. He was interviewed by Katz in 1974, and explained that he himself had no interest in changing his sexuality.[77] He had 17 shock treatments, and he vividly described the sense of disorientation following the treatments, as well as the fear the treatment aroused:

> I do remember after my own shock treatment listening to other people having shock treatment. I don't think that should be allowed. . . . You hear that horrible scream.[78]

Upon his release from the hospital, he told his mother he still didn't see anything wrong with his sexual preference, and she responded: "$62,000 for nothing! You haven't changed a bit."[79] In fact he had changed quite a bit—he experienced a great deal of memory loss. When he got home, he read his mail, and could not remember many of the people who wrote to him, including a lover who had clearly been special to him, though he added that his memory gradually returned over a period of several years.

Another case was that of Rick Stokes, a politician and gay rights activist who was a contemporary of Harvey Milk and who ran unsuccessfully against Milk for San Francisco supervisor in 1977.[80] His account is harrowing, and the ECT was not his idea, although he says he was cooperative because he was trying to become straight.[81] Stokes married in the hopes of changing his sexual orientation, a goal that was shared by his wife when she learned of it. His father-in-law was also deeply disturbed: "He was a strong man who had never had a son and I was his 'boy' . . ."[82] His in-laws then threatened his own parents, saying that if Stokes were not treated voluntarily in a sanitarium, they would commit him to the state hospital. Stokes was then 23. When he did go to the sanitarium, the doctor offered castration as a possible remedy, but offered to try other treatments first. Stokes said that calling the treatments frightening was "the understatement of the year."[83] He was unsure how many sessions he had, only able to estimate that it was between 10 and 50. At one point, he related:

> My mother had bought me a new watch . . . and I recall one time I had a treatment, and we forgot to take off the watch. We went to the jewelry store, and the watchmaker put the watch on whatever machine it was—he was trying to see what was wrong with it. The sparks flew from it—very visible sparks. The realization that this was happening to your brain while you were out made a real impression on me.[84]

Using ECT in an attempt to change sexuality is also one of the most blatant examples we have of ECT being used to enforce social norms, even in the absence of other "pathology." We know that some gay people, like Stokes, did internalize the idea that their sexuality was an illness.[85] But there is a powerful symbolism in how Liebman's patient, with whom we began the chapter, clearly cordoned off his psychosis, which he acknowledged as illness, from his sexuality, which he did not. It is to Liebman's credit that he clearly documented in a published report his patient's objections to having his sexuality medicalized.

We do not know how common it was to use ECT to treat homosexuality. Even if it was rare, though, the use of ECT to try to alter sexuality remains a disturbing aspect of ECT's history. Clinicians did believe they were genuinely treating an illness. This explains why none of the clinical depictions contain a hint of defensiveness. And some of the patients sought the treatment voluntarily. But there are important cautions to be learned here. One is that we should be wary of inventing illness categories out of behaviors, even if the intent is the laudable desire to reduce stigma. And we should be especially wary of applying highly invasive treatments with known risks when we do so.

This part of ECT's history also matters because, like other dismal aspects of the history, it has become a part of the social memory of the treatment. The image of ECT as a form of social coercion is one-sided, but it is by no means one with no historical basis.

The view that ECT was inherently punitive was so widespread that some thought this was the reason it worked. In the era when unmodified ECT was common, it was especially reasonable to see it as punitive. But the theory that this was the source of its efficacy had another foundation, namely psychoanalytic theories that a cause of mental illness was an overly punitive superego. The reasoning here was that externally applied punishment would relieve the superego of its duty to make the person suffer for unconscious guilt.

Medical theories influence patient experience of illness and treatment. Patients absorb perceptions of professional opinion (although those perceptions may sometimes be misperceptions), and this influences their interpretation of experience. Put more concretely, the belief that one's suffering is due to a traumatic life event or, by contrast, to a "chemical imbalance" has an effect on how one feels. Sylvia Plath, for example, had no access to theories of chemical imbalance, or genetic etiology. She certainly had life events that were traumatic for her, both in childhood and as an adult, and she saw them as the cause of her considerable anguish. She also believed that she had an overly punitive superego, and construed her improved mood after a short course of ECT as due to a need to be punished.

The history of psychoanalysis is rife with unfortunate tendencies to orthodoxy. Psychoanalytic reactions to convulsive therapy were, though, quite varied. Some advocates of somatic therapy cast psychoanalysts as their opponents from the start, but unequivocal opposition to somatic treatments was far from universal among psychoanalysts.

Notes

1 Samuel Liebman, "Homosexuality, Transvestism, and Psychosis: Study of a Case Treated with Electroshock," *Journal of Nervous and Mental Disease* 99 (1949) 945–958. The published description of the case actually suggests that the patient may have been having a manic episode, but this was not a diagnostic possibility Liebman seems to have pursued.
2 The use of ECT to treat homosexuality is covered in more detail later in this chapter.
3 Liebman, "Homosexuality, Transvestism, and Psychosis," 952.
4 Liebman, "Homosexuality, Transvestism, and Psychosis," 947.
5 Liebman, "Homosexuality, Transvestism, and Psychosis."
6 On the rise and fall of homosexuality as an illness category in American psychiatry, see Ronald Bayer, *Homosexuality and American Psychiatry* (Princeton: Princeton University Press, 1987).
7 Chauncey has argued that cross-dressing was more tolerated among working-class gay men, suggesting this may have been a concern about middle-class respectability for Liebman's patient. George Chauncey, *Gay New York: Gender,*

Urban Culture, and the Making of the Gay Male World, 1890–1940 (New York: Basic Books, 1994).

8 On the backlash, see Chauncey, *Gay New York* and David K. Johnson, *Lavender Scare: The Cold War Persecution of Gays and Lesbians in the Federal Government* (Chicago: University of Chicago Press, 2006). On the challenges one could face being both gay and African-American, see John D'Emilio, *Lost Prophet: The Life and Times of Bayard Rustin* (New York: The Free Press, 2003).

9 Thomas Szasz, *The Myth of Mental Illness: Foundations of a Theory of Personal Conduct* (New York: Harper Perennial, 2010, originally published 1961).

10 Peter Breggin, *Toxic Psychiatry: Why Therapy, Empathy, and Love Must Replace the Drugs, Electroshock, and Biochemical Theories* (New York: St. Martin's Griffin, 1994).

11 Braslow, *Mental Ills and Bodily Cures*, 106.

12 See the debate that ensued in the journal *History of Psychiatry* after the publication of Andrew Scull's "Psychiatry and Social Control in the Nineteenth and Twentieth Century," *History of Psychiatry* 2 (June 1991) 149–169.

13 George Makari, who is both a psychiatrist and a historian of psychiatry, has written an eloquent piece on how this tension has influenced his own work. George Makari, "Notes from Psychiatry's Battle Lines," *New York Times,* February 23, 2016.

14 Thomas Szasz is the exemplar here. I look at his ideas in more detail in Chapter Five.

15 Critical distinctions among different uses of the term were developed (rather brilliantly) by Ian Hacking in *The Social Construction of What?* (Cambridge: Harvard University Press, 2000).

16 Allen Horwitz, *The Logic of Social Control* (New York: Plenum Press, 1990), 9.

17 Talcott Parsons, "Social Structure and Dynamic Process: The Case of Modern Medical Practice," in *The Social System* (Glencoe: The Free Press, 1951), 428–479.

18 John C. Burnham, "Why Sociologists Abandoned the Sick Role Concept," *History of the Human Sciences* 27, 1 (2014) 70–87.

19 One of the best recent studies of this is Peter Conrad, *The Medicalization of Society: On the Transformation of Human Conditions into Treatable Diseases* (Baltimore: The Johns Hopkins University Press, 2007).

20 There are many accounts; for one, see Bayer, *Homosexuality and American Psychiatry*.

21 Sarah W. Tracy, *Alcoholism in America: From Reconstruction to Prohibition* (Baltimore: The Johns Hopkins University Press, 2005).

22 Gail Hornstein, *Agnes's Jacket: A Psychologist's Search for the Meanings of Madness* (New York: Rodale Books, 2009).

23 Norman S. Endler, *Holiday of Darkness: A Psychologist's Personal Journey Out of His Depression* (Toronto: John Wiley & Sons, Inc., 1982).

24 Endler, *Holiday of Darkness*, 65–66.

25 Peter G. Cranford, *But for the Grace of God: The Inside Story of the World's Largest Insane Asylum* (Augusta: Great Pyramid Press, 1981).

26 Shorter and Healy.

27 Cranford, *But for the Grace of God*, 88.

28 Cranford, *But for the Grace of God*, 88.

29 Cranford, *But for the Grace of God*, 88–89.

30 Cranford, *But for the Grace of God*, 86.

31 Milledgeville is pointed to as an unfortunate, but uncommon, abuse in Shorter and Healy, *Shock Therapy*, 93–94. They do not really establish empirically that Milledgeville was an outlier. They also say that this kind of abuse is outweighed by the number of people who have forfeited or been kept from helpful ECT treatment because of unfair stigma against it. Both numbers, however, are speculative.

32 Jonathan Metzl, *The Protest Psychosis: How Schizophrenia Became a Black Disease* (Boston: Beacon Press, 2009), 40.
33 Ivan Belknap, *Human Problems of a State Mental Hospital* (New York: McGraw-Hill Book Company, 1956), 164, 191.
34 Belknap, *Human Problems,* 191–192.
35 Belknap, *Human Problems,* 193.
36 Belknap, *Human Problems,* 193–194.
37 Belknap, *Human Problems,* 194.
38 Belknap, *Human Problems,* 194.
39 Joel Braslow, *Mental Ills and Bodily Cures.*
40 Belknap, *Human Problems,* 193.
41 Matthew Joseph Gambino, *Mental Health and Ideals of Citizenship: Patient Care at St. Elizabeth's Hospital in Washington, D.C., 1903–1962,* Ph. D. Dissertation, University of Illinois at Urbana-Champaign, 2010.
42 Gambino, *Mental Health and Ideals of Citizenship,* 166.
43 See, for example, J. Fremont Bateman and H. Warren Dunham, "The State Mental Hospital as a Specialized Community Experience," *American Journal of Psychiatry* 105, 6 (December 1948) 445–448.
44 Erving Goffman, *Asylums: Essays on the Social Situation of Mental Patients and Other Inmates* (Garden City: Anchor Books, 1961), 7.
45 Goffman, *Asylums,* 79.
46 Mary Jane Ward, "Out of the Dark Ages," *Woman's Home Companion,* August, 1946.
47 John Maurice Grimes, *When Minds Go Wrong: A Simple Story of the Mentally Ill—Past, Present, and Future* (Chicago: Published by the Author, 1949), 100.
48 Beam, *Gracefully Insane,* 154.
49 Kneeland and Warren, *Pushbutton Psychiatry,* 59. Kneeland and Warren looked at their sources for evidence of women being returned to the role of housewife, but they repeatedly omitted instances in those same sources where returning the women to their social roles meant returning her to work. They also repeatedly omitted any mention of the descriptions of illness in women patients, and so give the impression of doctors bent simply on making women into housewives, with no therapeutic intent involved.
50 There is not, and never has been, anything like a national database of ECT patients. The judgment that the majority have been women has been made by numerous observers, based on casual observation as well as the incomplete figures that appeared in published studies. It is probably a correct judgment, but it remains an educated guess, not an empirically established fact.
51 See my review of Kneeland and Warren, *Pushbutton Psychiatry,* in the *Bulletin of the History of Medicine* 77 (2003) 471–472.
52 Braslow, *Mental Ills and Bodily Cures,* 119–123.
53 Paul Popenoe, *Marriage Is What You Make It* (New York: The MacMillan Company, 1950), 124, cited in Kneeland and Warren, *Pushbutton Psychiatry,* 60.
54 N. K. Rickles and Charles G. Polan, "Causes of Failure in Treatment with Electric Shock: Analysis of Thirty-Eight Cases," *Archives of Neurology and Psychiatry* 59 (1948) 337–346, cited in Kneeland and Warren, *Pushbutton Psychiatry,* 59.
55 Rickles and Polan, "Causes of Failure," 339.
56 Julius I. Steinfeld, *Therapeutic Studies on Psychotics: A Psychological and Psychosomatic Approach in Four Papers* (Des Plaines, IL: Forest Press Publishers, 1951). This is one of the sources cited in Kneeland and Warren, *Pushbutton Psychiatry,* but the authors drew on only one of many cases discussed in the book, and divorced their discussion of even that case from the context of the multifaceted treatment plan Steinfeld was describing.

57 Steinfeld's study includes many more case histories of women than of men: by my count, 33 women and only 6 men. Kneeland and Warren, conceding that a chapter on the treatment of postpartum illness was of necessity limited to a study of women, note that one other chapter names only one male patient, but that simply amounts to leaving out the other chapters where male patients are discussed. Kneeland and Warren, *Pushbutton Psychiatry,* 59.
58 Steinfeld, *Therapeutic Studies on Psychotics,* 22.
59 Kneeland and Warren, *Pushbutton Psychiatry,* 59.
60 Judith Kruger, *My Fight for Sanity* (Greenwich: Crest Books, 1959). I thank Jennifer Tomich for this reference.
61 Kruger, *My Fight for Sanity,* 7–9.
62 Kruger, *My Fight for Sanity,* 9.
63 Kruger, *My Fight for Sanity,* 55.
64 Kruger, *My Fight for Sanity,* 55.
65 Kruger, *My Fight for Sanity,* 55.
66 Stanley Joel Reiser, *Medicine and the Reign of Technology* (Cambridge: Cambridge University Press, 1981).
67 Kruger, *My Fight for Sanity,* 232–233.
68 Kruger, *My Fight for Sanity,* 140.
69 Kruger, *My Fight for Sanity,* 78.
70 See Bayer, *Homosexuality and American Psychiatry,* on the challenge to psychiatry's definition of homosexuality as an illness, and the profession's response.
71 On both of these points, see George Chauncey, *Gay New York.*
72 See Johnson, *The Lavender Scare.*
73 Jennifer Terry, *An American Obsession: Science, Medicine, and Homosexuality in Modern Society* (Chicago: University of Chicago Press, 1999), 69–70.
74 Newdigate M. Owensby, "Homosexuality and Lesbianism Treated with Metrazol: A Preliminary Report," *Journal of Nervous and Mental Diseases* 92 (July 1940) 65–66.
75 George N. Thompson, "Electroshock and other Therapeutic Considerations in Sexual Psychopathy," *Journal of Nervous and Mental Disease* 109 (1949) 531–539.
76 Jonathan Katz, *Gay American History: Lesbians and Gay Men in the U.S.A.* (New York: Thomas Y. Crowell, 1976).
77 Katz, *Gay American History,* 201.
78 Katz, *Gay American History,* 203–204.
79 Katz, *Gay American History,* 204–205.
80 Stokes's experience with ECT is described in Nancy Adair and Casey Adair, *Word is Out: Stories of Some of Our Lives* (New York: Dell Publishing Co., 1978), 34–36.
81 Adair and Adair, *Word is Out,* 36.
82 Adair and Adair, *Word is Out,* 34.
83 Adair and Adair, *Word is Out,* 34.
84 Adair and Adair, *Word is Out,* 35. It is actually physically unlikely that sparks flew from a watch because of ECT.
85 This is explored in depth in Martin Duberman's autobiography, *Cures: A Gay Man's Odyssey* (Cambridge, MA: Westview Press, 2002, originally published 1992).

4 "What of His Psychology?"

ECT and Psychoanalysis

"'What of his psychology?' . . . 'Absolutely of no importance!'"

One of the great classics of post–World War II American fiction depicts electroconvulsive therapy (ECT) as a form of discipline for the protagonist. While the treatment is administered, a doctor explains that the treatment will not only benefit the patient, but society as well, once the patient is subdued. What is striking to the reader, though, is that the "patient" depicted seems to show no signs of real psychopathology. Rather, the ECT is administered purely as a form of social control. This is, of course, a classic storyline of the antipsychiatry movement, and the description so far could describe that movement's famous literary representation, *One Flew Over the Cuckoo's Nest*. I refer, though, to Ralph Ellison's *Invisible Man,* a work that predates most of the key texts of the antipsychiatry movement, and appeared in the early days of ECT.[1] The medical procedure in *Invisible Man* is as unnamed as the protagonist, but it is unmistakably ECT—he is "pumped between live electrodes like an accordion," his head "encircled by a piece of cold metal like the iron cap worn by the occupant of an electric chair."[2] He also experiences some short-term memory loss, a common side effect of ECT.

In an evocation of the objectification the Invisible Man experiences at other points in the novel, the doctors talk about him and his treatment as if he is not there. They debate among themselves the humaneness of the procedure, one of them comparing it with unease to lobotomy. The more enthusiastic doctor praises the treatment, responding to the question "What of his psychology?" with "Absolutely of no importance!. . . . The patient will live as he has to live, and with absolute integrity. Who could ask more? He'll experience no major conflict of motives, and what is even better, society will suffer no traumata on his account."[3]

Ellison published *Invisible Man* in 1947, nine years after the invention of ECT, and in this scene captures a debate within the psychiatric profession, between those who saw shock treatments in psychiatry as a major scientific advance for psychiatry, and those who worried that their success would encourage inattention to psychological dimensions of patients. Ellison's success in rendering a debate within the psychiatric profession might be partly attributable to his short experience working part-time for Harry Stack Sullivan, a psychiatrist who was among the most vehemently opposed to somatic treatments.[4] Ellison's depiction describes a continuing tension within the psychiatric profession between the somatic and psychological approaches, one with obvious resonances for the present state of psychiatry. This tension is often rendered by the common historical metaphor of the pendulum. In this rendering, we view psychiatry as swinging back and forth between the two poles represented by the doctors in overseeing the Invisible Man's ECT. The pendulum metaphor is ubiquitous in discussions of psychiatry's history, and may in fact dominate our understanding of that history.[5]

Yet as much as Ellison's fiction captured a truth about psychiatric controversy, it is equally crucial to see that the dialogue shows the two clinicians working together, and sharing one another's assumptions. The biological psychiatrist adopts the psychoanalytic view that inner conflict could be a source of nervous morbidity. The psychological psychiatrist does not question the efficacy of the procedure, but asks more modestly whether it omits an important dimension of treatment. This sharing of assumptions is in fact more reflective of the reality of psychiatry's history than the polarized picture we often receive.

This chapter has two goals, one empirical and one theoretical. The empirical goal is to examine the response of American psychoanalysis to the introduction of ECT, as a case study for understanding the complex interactions between psychological and somatic approaches. The theoretical goal is to assess what is gained and what is lost by interpreting the history of psychiatry through the pendulum metaphor. The two goals are related because the pendulum metaphor—probably the dominant metaphor in psychiatric historiography—is poorly suited to capturing the complexities of the interactions between approaches.[6]

The pendulum metaphor is not so much wrong as incomplete. It does capture aspects of the history of psychiatry. And my objection is not that it *is* a metaphor; metaphors are essential for making very complex phenomena, such as the history of a profession, intelligible. In this case, however, the intelligibility comes at the cost of obscuring critical nuances in the development of American psychiatry. The weakness of the pendulum metaphor is that it is a "dead" metaphor—that is, one whose status as metaphor may sometimes be forgotten.[7] It can lead historians to caricature eras in psychiatric history.

PSYCHIATRY'S "INNER CONFLICT"

According to some contemporary rhetoric, as the twenty-first century dawns, immediately following the decade of the brain, developments in our knowledge of neuroscience promise to render our psychiatry truly scientific at last. Our growing understanding of genetics offers hope for a more certain understanding of the etiology of mental illness, and so will lift the stigma attached to the mentally ill. Our knowledge of the specific functions of the regions of the brain grows yearly, promising a similar specificity in therapeutics. Our theories of mental illness are being sifted from the mists of philosophy and grounded in the solid sciences of biology and chemistry.

And yet, almost identical rhetoric dominated the close of the nineteenth century. As Nathan Hale has commented on neurologists' mood in the last decades of the nineteenth century, "It is difficult to exaggerate the neurologists' sense of expectancy, their faith that within the foreseeable future every puzzle would be solved at last."[8]

Professions may be defined as much by their perennial inner conflicts as by their overtly stated missions. The profession of psychiatry has shown over its history a continual tension between the "somatic" (or bodily) style on the one hand, and the more strictly psychological modes of treatment of the talk therapies.[9] This reflects a debate over how best to relieve the suffering of the mentally ill, which is of course psychiatry's distinctive mission.

Consider several quotations which, taken together, embody psychiatry's inner friction. A pair of psychiatrists wrote the first over half a century ago, but one can easily imagine the same quote appearing in a psychiatric journal today, with modest changes in diction:

> Doubts and misgivings assail the contemporary psychiatrist regarding the importance of psychological or biological factors in the etiology of functional psychoses, and psychological or pharmacological methods in their treatment.[10]

Or consider the uneasiness expressed about the rising importance of physiological treatments in this statement from two psychiatrists in 1943:

> One of the less fortunate consequences of such impersonal pharmacologic and physical methods of treatment has been a loss of interest not only in the problems of psychopathology and psychogenesis but also in those of psychotherapy.[11]

At the time these were written, Sullivan was a prominent advocate of a more strictly psychological approach. One of America's leading psychiatrists at mid-century, Sullivan wrote:

> I refer here to the Freeman lobotomy, the metrazol and camphor convulsive treatments, the electroshock. . . . These sundry procedures, to my way of thinking, produce 'beneficial' results by reducing the patient's capacity for being human. The philosophy is something to the effect that it is better to be a contented imbecile than a schizophrenic.[12]

To Sullivan, biological psychiatry was effective, but only in a cruel way. But as one of his contemporaries countered,

> Who is the more sadistic, the psychotherapist who permits a patient to suffer torture while undergoing months or years of treatment for a depression, or the psychiatrist who, using convulsive therapy, enables him to regain his peace of mind and feelings of well-being in at most a few weeks?[13]

The discord reflected in these quotes is in evidence today, as psychiatrists and laypeople react with enthusiasm, uneasy acceptance, or dismay to the current boom in psychopharmacology. Many react to this tension as if it were newly existing, but it is an enduring and repetitive conflict.

This sense of repetition tempers my agreement with anthropologist T. M. Luhrmann's description of a "growing disorder in American psychiatry."[14] But it is true that the resurgence of biological or "somatic" psychiatry increasingly marginalizes the talk therapies. Many have called for an integrated or holistic psychiatry—what is sometimes called a biopsychosocial approach—but these voices have frequently seemed faint, drowned out by the insistence that only one approach is truly efficacious and humane.

The quote from Sullivan might seem a typical psychoanalytic response, and more than one commentator has cited it as an example of prejudice, a knee-jerk response of a talk therapist to an effective treatment that did not fit his paradigm.[15] But his comments on somatic treatments have been cited more frequently than he likely expected, a point I return to below. To treat it as representative of psychoanalytic thought is very misleading.

Psychoanalytic Reactions to the Introduction of ECT

As we have seen, there were many reasons for the rapid spread of ECT in the United States in its early years. Yet Shorter has proposed that it might have been welcomed even more robustly were it not for theoretical prejudice:

> ECT did not have a truly triumphal march in the United States. For one thing, the psychoanalysts were generally opposed to it. . . . Throughout the American psychoanalytic literature ran a begrudging suspiciousness of electroshock. This was combined with an insistence that ECT's utility must rest on some kind of psychodynamic basis rather than on brain biology. For if the neurons of the brain itself were making people ill, the theoretical structure of psychoanalysis flew out the window.[16]

According to Shorter, then, the psychoanalysts opposed and misrepresented ECT, because of the threat it represented to their paradigm. This view of the psychoanalytic response to ECT is partly accurate. Some suspicion there was, and psychoanalytic explanations for ECT's efficacy often did suggest psychodynamic reasons. But published clinical reports also show that few psychoanalysts saw psychological and physiological interpretations as incompatible. And the range and flexibility of psychoanalytic views of ECT were greater than has been suggested.

Although historians and psychiatrists have sometimes blamed Freud—with some justification—for diverting psychiatry from biology, Freud believed that biological research would eventually confirm his theories. In other words, while he believed that that his theories were psychologically demonstrable, he never denied that there was a neurochemistry of the mind, and was deeply materialist in many of his assumptions.[17]

Freud never wrote about ECT; he died the year after it was invented. In his discussion of war neuroses, he did add an appendix on non-convulsive electrical treatment that may have influenced later psychoanalytic under-standings of ECT.[18] Freud believed that electric shocks for war neurosis were effective because they reversed the flight into illness caused by combat into a flight into health, away from the intentionally painful treatment. In other words, he saw it as a ruthless elimination of the secondary gain from war neurosis. He added that this treatment "bore a stigma from the outset. It did not aim at the patient's recovery, or not in the first instance; it aimed, above all, at restoring his fitness for service. Here Medicine was serving purposes foreign to its essence."[19] He concluded, not surprisingly, that the treatment did not bring about lasting cure. This was consistent with the psychoanalytic dictum that no treatment that failed to work through unconscious conflict would provide lasting results for neurosis. He also argued that late in the war, the current was increased to very cruel levels in German hospitals, due to what he regarded as a peculiarly German ten-dency "to carry through . . . intentions regardless of all else."[20]

This use of electricity in military psychiatry usually had a clinical ratio-nale quite different from that of convulsive therapy. Physicians used it in a combination of suggestion, exploiting patients' magical beliefs in the heal-ing powers of electricity, as well as the aversive conditioning that troubled Freud.[21] In a sense, despite the direct application of electricity to the body, this was more a psychological form of treatment than a somatic one. It probably, however, influenced many later understandings of ECT.[22] As late as the 1960s, when psychoanalytic interpretations of ECT's efficacy were already losing some influence, a major author in the antipsychiatry move-ment described ECT's efficacy as a form of suggestion in terms very similar to those used by the military psychiatrists during World War I.[23]

There is no question that Freud's followers have often resisted somatic thera-pies, and this did influence responses to ECT. Smith Ely Jelliffe, for example, was an early critic of lobotomy, a procedure he likened to "burning down the house to roast a pig."[24] But the psychoanalytic reaction to ECT was far from monolithic, ranging from those who were deeply hostile, to those who con-ceded efficacy but discouraged the practice for reasons of safety, to those who positively saw convulsion therapies as a useful adjunct to insight-oriented talk therapies. Sullivan's view was not in fact typical of analysts, and Otto Fenichel, author of one of the most influential psychoanalytic books in America, described

Sullivan's view as radical.[25] Psychoanalytic responses to ECT included theoretical prejudice, but also reasoned caution and outright support.

Braslow points out: "Since it acted on the body, one would assume that electroconvulsive therapy reinforced physicians' belief in an organically based model of psychiatric illness."[26] Such was the power of psychoanalytic thought at mid-century, however, that even a surgical intervention like lobotomy was understood by some in psychoanalytic terms. Noting that many fretful patients became calm and contented immediately following a lobotomy, many psychiatrists in the 1940s—and not just analysts—believed that the removal of the frontal lobes in lobotomy was in effect an excision of the overly punitive superego that was the cause of the psychiatric symptoms.[27]

There were related understandings of ECT. Some analysts saw the use of ECT as a form of sadism, representing unconscious hostility to the mentally ill. Fenichel analyzed doctors who applied shock, and found that they had feelings (conscious or unconscious) of killing the patients and bringing them back to life. Gregory Zilboorg, the well-known psychiatrist who was also a historian of medicine, was a prominent example of a psychoanalyst who shared Sullivan's hostility to the use of somatic therapies. Zilboorg thought convulsive therapies enacted a "repetition compulsion" through which physicians acted out a desire to punish the patient for having an illness that frightened the doctor.[28] But any imagined punitive aspect to ECT was not necessarily, in psychoanalytic thought, an argument against using it. In fact, for some analysts, the punishment was the mechanism of efficacy. As Braslow put it, in this theory "the patient experiences the treatment as a sadistic punishing attack which satisfies his unconscious sense of guilt, obviating the need for self-punishment."[29]

This view of ECT developed in part from earlier interpretations of other forms of shock and convulsive treatment. An important source for this was a study conducted in Baltimore's Enoch Pratt Hospital by psychoanalyst Edith Weigert, published in 1940, and cited by many later psychoanalytic authors on ECT.[30] Weigert studied patients treated with Metrazol and prolonged narcosis. She concluded that convulsion therapies acted as substitute superegos. Beyond its importance as an influence, there are two points worth noting about Weigert's study. One is that her argument had some plausibility based on her patients' experiences. Several of them did come into treatment tormented by feelings of guilt, and many reported deep relief from these feelings following the treatment—although in several cases that feeling did not last. Weigert, though, did not show that the patients did in fact experience the treatment as punitive; she seems to have assumed that anyone would regard such treatments as threatening, if not outright sadistic. She also did not consider that the guilt could have been alleviated as the result of the depression lifting, instead of the reverse.

Secondly, while Weigert was advancing a psychoanalytic interpretation of the somatic therapies, she was not hostile to the somatic therapies, nor was she trying to deny that convulsive therapy worked on the body. On the contrary, she explicitly argued that the choice between a physical and a psychological theory was a false one.[31] Weigert cited Adolf Meyer and other American psychiatrists who viewed mental illness as disturbances to "the psychobiological entity"—in everyday language, the whole person. It is remarkable that this view—seemingly so reasonable, and articulated by so prominent a figure as Meyer—has been so often marginalized in psychiatric rhetoric.

Psychoanalyst Eric Mosse advanced similar ideas to Weigert's in articles published in the mid-1940s that focused more on ECT itself.[32] Mosse, noting the rapid spread of ECT in American hospitals, thought physicians were showing an almost magical faith in it. Mosse was very confident that ECT acted psychosomatically, although in an earlier article written with John Millet, he was more open to considering, as they put it, that "psyche and soma" acted in concert.[33] He also lamented that few psychiatrists were taking into account the psychology of the experience of shock. He criticized his colleagues for leaving the room during the period of disorientation following the application of the treatment, arguing that this state offers the best opportunity for psychological observation. Organically minded clinicians, he believed, had attributed differences in convulsion types to technical details such as differences in the current applied, the placement of the electrodes, the thickness of the skull, or even the weather. Mosse believed that a key and ignored variable was the patient's degree of psychological resistance, and he claimed to have frequently observed a "masochistic eagerness" of the patient to undergo the treatment. For such a patient, "his craving for atonement to ease his guilt will keep the threshold lower than in others where aggression, anxiety and stubbornness are deep-rooted and outstanding trends of their neurosis."[34]

Mosse's views were all plausible from within the frame of psychoanalytic assumptions, but his data are also subject to plausible re-readings by those who do not share those assumptions. His interpretations now read like blunt impositions of psychoanalytic templates, but they were offered with all the confidence psychoanalysis's mid-century prestige provided. Mosse, for example, cited a woman who believed that the doctor was the devil, or that the devil was inside her in the shape of a pig, and he claimed that "behind these phantasies was the patient's struggle against her instinctual drives toward her father." More time and voltage became necessary to achieve the *grand mal,* and at the same time "a mild grade of stubbornness rose sharply to a high pitch of obstinacy." This, Mosse believed, was evidence that the patient was re-enacting the struggle with her father with the doctor. Mosse also claimed that in the 10–30 minutes following the treatment, patients were in a state of regression, "thrown back in a state of earliest infancy where those phenomena and mechanisms come to an unchecked appearance which evidently presented the leading conflict with the super-ego."[35] He cited in this respect one patient whose professional "success was blocked by masochistic and self-punishing behavior, behavior that compromised his psychoanalysis as well":

Although the paranoid, sado-masochistic character of the superficially quiet, polite and anxious patient was here already established, it needed the spectacular reaction in the *psychological shock-situation* to reveal the depths of these trends. The patient would shout for over half an hour on top of his voice: 'Mother, mother, mother, mother,' struggling, fighting, shouting and crying to such an extent that special strapping devices became necessary to keep the patient on the table.[36]

Mosse's account of this patient does not really establish paranoia or sado-masochism, although these may have been present. By stressing the patient's psychodynamics above all, it minimizes reference to the objectively frightening character of the treatment.

Mosse claimed to have found that in over half of the patients he observed the gag seemed to be experienced as the nipple of the mother's breast. He cited as evidence the sucking at the gag, and the unwillingness to allow the gag to be removed:

The time until the patient finally lets go could be looked upon as being in direct proportion to the strength of his oral fixation. A few minutes later, this type of patient would often sit up cuddling his face on the breast of the attending nurse, looking at her with the expression of ecstatic love and erotic enthrallment.[37]

Mosse also considered patients who did not benefit from shock treatment, such as this one:

One of these patients, a middle-aged woman who didn't want anything else but childish attention, could not be helped by any of her some 20 previous doctors, because any 'cure' would have deprived her of further attention and worry, especially from her neurotic, 18-year-old son. It was the replica of her behavior in childhood toward a father whom she had tried to castrate through all her life by this demanding 'sickness.' Each time when she was lying prepared for the shock treatment, with the electrodes fixed to her temples, she would remark with a smile: 'Do you really think that this is going to help me?' Of course, it didn't; ridiculing and raving about the quacks and inefficiency of doctors, she would 'desperately' proceed to castrate the next doctor.[38]

In the same issue of the journal where this article by Mosse appeared, one psychiatrist critical of Mosse accused him of grafting psychoanalytic ideas onto "a wholly new treatment."[39] Accepting Mosse's interpretations does require faith in many of his assumptions; he certainly did not provide much corroborative evidence for them. But while he unquestionably adopted a psychoanalytic paradigm, that paradigm did not cause him to reduce the mechanism of efficacy for ECT to psychological causes. He, like Weigert, explicitly stressed that a relationship between mind and body should be assumed. Mosse was by no means hostile to ECT, but openly regarded it as a useful adjunct to psychotherapy. He in fact mentioned patients whose psychotherapeutic progress had been stalled, who were able to make significant progress after the ECT.

In the article Mosse wrote with Millet, they stated that many patients were openly or secretly eager for the treatment—leaving the reader to wonder how they knew this about the ones for whom it was secret. This eagerness had several sources, they thought: magical thinking in patients who longed for an omnipotent father for some; the desire for attention—patients observed correctly that ECT patients received a lot of attention from the clinical staff; and in "some instances the gratification anticipated is of a clearly masochistic character." They unequivocally asserted the efficacy of the treatment, calling it an "invaluable" adjunct to psychotherapy, still regarding the latter as essential to lasting recovery. Note the enthusiasm in this passage:

> One of the most satisfying of the observations to be made in connection with recovery following electroshock treatment is the obvious return of self-confidence, initiative and impatience to get back to life. Profound discouragement disappears, doubt of the physician's ability to help is replaced by gratitude and confidence . . . Under the impact of this newfound psychic security the patient is often able to face and understand trends in his personality which previously he had shunned, or had evaluated as irremediable, and to look upon them as obstacles which could be overcome or reduced to minor significance.[40]

They proceeded to present a number of dramatic cases of recovery in patients for whom psychotherapy had been stalled. Millet and Mosse did not seek to reduce the efficacy of ECT to psychological mechanisms; in fact, they explicitly warned against posing a false choice between "psyche" and "soma." While reiterating the view that convulsive therapy was perceived as punitive for at least some patients, they also proposed that

> experimental neuro-physiologists have demonstrated that associations of recent origin are more easily broken down by reconditioning procedures than those which have been long established. The same principle is observed in operation in the course of any psychoanalytic treatment. Violent interruption of the associative pathways, therefore, would seem to topple the structure of pathological superimposed associations and to reinstate the more orderly pattern of associations through which the mastery of reality is achieved.[41]

So, in this understanding, just as one can expect a physiological intervention such as ECT to have psychological benefits, a talk therapy is expected to have physiological effects.

The notion that patients experienced ECT as punitive was not simply a theoretical assertion, but one several researchers thought was grounded empirically. Several researchers found patients fearful of ECT (as many patients continue to be today). Some patients reported feelings of going through something like a near-death experience, and rebirth: "It changes my body like magic," "It makes me unconscious and I awaken like new," and "It rejuvenates me, uses me up and makes me into a different person" were some of the descriptions by patients.[42]

These studies of subjective response provided little evidence that patients experienced the treatment as a punishment. This is probably not because such evidence was hard to come by, but rather because the authors thought it too obvious to require proof. By far the majority of accounts of ECT in its early years, whether by clinicians or patients, describe it as terrifying, and patients often experienced it as punitive regardless of clinical intent, even when they acknowledged therapeutic benefits. This sense that a procedure so terrible must be punitive was well captured, for example, in Sylvia Plath's *The Bell Jar*. The narrator, Esther Greenwood (who is usually taken to be an alter ego for Plath), comments after an ECT treatment: "I wondered what terrible thing it was that I had done."[43]

There is little evidence that ECT's use was hindered by conceptual biases of the psychoanalytic establishment.[44] The Sullivan quote, about making patients of somatic psychiatry into contented imbeciles, is often adduced, but it actually appears in a *footnote* in Sullivan's published lectures, *Conceptions of Modern Psychiatry*—an obscure place to be leading a psychoanalytic charge against ECT. Some analysts, such as Fenichel, themselves regarded Sullivan's views as radical. Sullivan's stated views on somatic treatments, including ECT, say less about psychoanalytic assumptions than they do his own experience as a mental patient, and his feeling of relief that he was not subjected to somatic treatments that were unquestionably frightening to observers. Perry notes that when Sullivan "spoke of his own schizophrenic illness, he stated angrily that if electroshock or lobotomy had been in use in hospitals when he was growing up, he would have ended up his life as a 'vegetable.'"[45]

Any psychoanalytic doubts there were about ECT were abetted by a fact no clinician doubted: ECT was risky when first introduced. A recent clinical handbook of ECT use in fact claims that "modern ECT is so far removed from that primitive procedure [introduced in Rome in 1938] that it should hardly be considered the same treatment."[46] Amid all the controversies that have surrounded ECT, not even its most ardent supporters have ever questioned that it was a frightening and risky procedure in its early years. It was reasonable, then, for analysts to promote alternatives.

The openness of some psychoanalysts to somatic approaches was mirrored in the early years of ECT by openness to psychological views by clinicians with a more somatic emphasis. This openness of the "somaticists" may be less surprising, as this was the heyday of psychoanalysis. But it is still worth showing, in order to deepen appreciation of the extent of eclecticism in American psychiatry. This theoretical openness is evident, for example, in Lothar Kalinowsky and Paul Hoch's *Shock Treatments,* an important textbook from 1946 on somatic therapies.[47] *Shock Treatments* covers both chemical and electric convulsive therapies, as well as insulin coma therapy. The authors' leanings toward the somatic style was signaled in an etiological claim in the first sentence: "Psychological disorders like physical diseases are due to natural causes . . ."[48] Yet on the next page, Kalinowsky and Hoch made it clear that they accepted psychological modes of treatment, and that there were dangers in becoming overly preoccupied with the somatic aspects. They wrote, "The path between the 'organic' and 'psychological' extremes seems to hold the most promise for the future. . . . The effect of the shock therapies has encouraged many workers to overemphasize the 'organic' aspects [of mental illness] . . ."

Kalinowsky and Hoch were skeptical toward psychoanalytic theories of ECT's means of efficacy. They did not reject them on principle, but thought they were unsupported empirically. They pointed out, for example, that not all patients seemed to fear shock treatments, and that there was no statistical correlation between fearing the treatment and obtaining symptom relief.[49] But they were also open to the possibility that psychotherapy might be a useful adjunct to somatic treatments.[50] Presumably, if they had been asked of a patient, "What of his psychology?" they would not have answered that it was "of no importance."

Psychoanalytic theories of ECT's efficacy were still being cited in the 1970s.[51] Although they had always had their detractors, they lost favor less because they were explicitly refuted than because they fit more poorly with the evolving climate of psychiatry. The demonstration, in the late 1950s, that convulsion was necessary to have therapeutic effects undercut most of the psychological theories, because those theories had rarely suggested that convulsion was necessary to produce the sense of being punished.[52] More recently, the demonstration that real ECT outperforms sham ECT in clinical trials also weakens psychological theories.[53] But while there is some scientific basis for it, the decline of psychological theorizing about ECT is in important ways also a matter of fashion. Recent textbooks and clinical handbooks of ECT concede that the mechanism of efficacy is poorly under- stood, but entirely lack discussions of psychological theories. In a provoca- tive passage of *The Creation of Psychopharmacology,* Healy writes that "in the 1960s a new biomedical self was being born, entailing a significant series of consequences for how we understand and indeed experience ourselves."[54] Within that understanding and experience, psychological theories of ECT's efficacy may seem quaint.

But whether those theories have been superseded for scientific reasons or reasons of cultural climate, they need to be understood historically in their complexity. We have now recognized, after reading Pressman, that the depiction of the discarded therapy lobotomy *purely* as barbarism or social control is inadequate. Discarded psychoanalytic views of ECT merit analogous redemption from the condescension of posterity. Although they shared certain key assumptions, especially the view of the treatment as punitive, psychoanalytic authors differed on a number of key points. Those who were deeply opposed to all somatic treatments seem to have been a minority, and a minority that was openly censured for dogmatism by some colleagues. Opposition there was, and Millet and Mosse in fact wondered if it had an unconscious source in analysts' fear toward a potential threat to their livelihood.[55] And some psychoanalytic writers were positively enthusiastic about ECT—even if they tended to a psychological interpretation of its efficacy. Psychoanalysts, to be sure, saw ECT through psychoanalytic lenses. Those lenses did not lead to unified hostility to ECT, or to dogmatic rejection of somatic assumptions.

Beyond the Metaphor of the Pendulum

The view that the history of psychiatry is well represented by a pendulum metaphor is so common it may have the appearance of common sense. It is unlikely that it could become so ingrained if it were utterly fallacious. But when metaphors for historical processes do become so ingrained, they warrant scrutiny, and careful attention to what aspects of history they capture poorly. I believe there are at least four reasons we should be wary of uncritical uses of this particular metaphor.

One is that it may conceal continuity, the ways past approaches might survive, either explicitly or implicitly, into changing eras. Metzl, for example, has made a powerful argument for the unintended survival of psychoanalytic cultural habits into the era of psychopharmacology.[56] A second reason is that the metaphor of the pendulum lacks explanatory power. A pendulum swings because it follows laws of physics, but there is no obvious and necessary reason why clinical styles (or other historical phenomena, such as political leanings) should "swing." If in fact they do change in ways that seem well captured by the metaphor, we may wish to direct our research attention to explaining why that should be, instead of operating from an implicit assumption that that is how history works. Thirdly, the use of the pendulum metaphor risks reducing clinical and scientific change to mere fashion. Scientific fashion can, of course, be a factor in shaping the production of knowledge; it helps to set priorities for research agendas, and has deep influences in how data are interpreted. But it cannot explain everything. While the revival of ECT since the early 1980s is surely related to the revival of biological psychiatry in general, that change in fashion fails to explain some aspects of ECT's re-emergence. Why have certain somatic treatments fared better than others? Why, for example, has ECT seen a revival that has not been shared by other somatic treatments that were discontinued, such as insulin coma therapy and lobotomy? And why has ECT so often outperformed antidepressants in clinical trials? These questions cannot be answered simply by saying psychiatrists now have a somatic bias, an answer that ignores the scientific data showing ECT to be safe and effective. Historians can and should subject those data to critical analysis, but simply dismissing them as a product of our somatic times does not take us very far.

This chapter speaks most directly, though, to the fourth reason the pendulum metaphor is misleading. If we see psychiatry as swinging back and forth between two extremes, we will miss the extent of eclecticism and pragmatism present in any period, and risk exaggerating the dogmatism held by proponents of either style of psychiatry. This is not to deny that both sides have had their dogmatic reductionists. But if we see psychiatry as swinging back and forth between extremes represented by extremists, we will miss the enormous extent to which American psychiatrists have mixed styles in their pursuit of relief for their patients' pain. Most of the biological treatments—discarded ones such lobotomy, insulin coma therapy, and chemical convulsion therapy, as well as extant ones such as the early antipsychotics and antidepressants, and ECT—were developed during the period when psychodynamic theory was at its peak of influence.

There is some reason to think the pendulum metaphor for psychiatry's history developed from within the psychiatric profession itself[57] This could itself be considered a reason for historians to question it. Historians of psychiatry have too often re-enacted the polarities within psychiatry itself. To the extent that we continue to do so, we risk being unduly controlled by our object of study.

Psychoanalysis and ECT appear to many to be opposites in psychological medicine. And for good reason. Psychoanalysis is the archetypal talk therapy, ECT an iconic somatic treatment. ECT is fast acting, psychoanalysis a lengthy procedure. Psychoanalysis aims at the retrieval of memory, ECT threatens its loss.

Yet there are unexpected ways in which the two might be secret sharers. Both involve the patient assuming a supine position, with the loss of control and assertion that implies. This may seem superficial, but it is symbolic of a more significant similarity—both (when voluntary) require patients to take a radical leap of faith and assume the clinicians know what they are doing. Radical, because these are both very counter-intuitive treatments. From a narrow biomedical perspective it is as far out of "common sense" to free associate in the presence of a healer you cannot see, and who is bid to withhold most of the normal supports people offer one another in response to distress, as it is to most people to induce use electricity to induce convulsions. And radical too, in that the frequency of sessions, and length, and cost, of the process in psychoanalysis will normally seem like a big risk to take for many people seeking help. Here, as with ECT, many are likely to give it a try when less radical interventions have been found wanting. And radical, because there remains an element of mystery as to why they work, although practitioners of both are ardent that they do. This mystery, in turn, is abetted by the ways these two treatments, for very different reasons, are resistant to study by the methods of randomized controlled trials that are the gold standard for medical efficacy.

The radical leap, though, has always been one taken voluntarily by psychoanalytic patients. The same has not been true for ECT, and in the 1960s, as many forms of social authority came under question, psychiatry faced serious questioning about its practices, from both within and outside the profession. Involuntary and somatic treatments would come under especially harsh fire, and ECT was emblematic of both.

Acknowledgments

An earlier version of this chapter was published as "Beyond the Metaphor of the Pendulum: Electroconvulsive Therapy, Psychoanalysis, and the Styles of American Psychiatry," *The Journal of the History of Medicine and Allied Sciences* 61 (January, 2006) 1–25. This revision is published here with the permission of Oxford University Press.

Notes

1 Ralph Ellison, *Invisible Man* (New York: Vintage, 1990, originally published 1947), 236. I am grateful to Susan Reverby for conversations and correspondence that deepened my understanding of Ellison's work.
2 Ellison, *Invisible Man,* 232–233.
3 Ellison, *Invisible Man,* 236. This depiction of ECT fits a pattern set in other episodes of *Invisible Man.* Much of the novel is about the shallow benevolence the protagonist encounters from white society, from liberal paternalists and white Marxists, among others, and this seems to be embodied in this medical encounter, too.
4 Helen Swick Perry, *Psychiatrist of America: The Life of Harry Stack Sullivan* (Cambridge: The Belknap Press of Harvard University Press, 1982), 348–349. Sullivan shared his work with Ellison, seeking help with his writing.
5 Examples of the explicit use of the pendulum metaphor to describe the history of psychiatry include J. Allan Hobson and Jonathan A. Leonard, *Out of Its Mind: Psychiatry in Crisis* (Cambridge, MA: Perseus Publishing, 2001), 220; Don R. Lipsitt, "Psyche and Soma: Struggles to Close the Gap," in Roy W. Menninger and John C. Nemiah, eds., *American Psychiatry after World War II* (Washington, DC: American Psychiatric Press, 2000), 154; and Glen Gabbard, *The Psychology of the Sopranos: Love, Death, Desire and Betrayal in America's Favorite Gangster Family* (New York: Basic Books, 2002), 21. Lipsitt's chapter points out that amid every swing of the pendulum, there have been contrary currents. Using the word "cycle" instead of "pendulum," Mark S. Micale also represents psychiatry's history as an alternation between extremes, in "The Psychiatric Body," in Roger 344.
6 This chapter is adapted from my 2006 article, "Beyond the Metaphor of the Pendulum: Electroconvulsive Therapy, Psychoanalysis, and the Styles of American Psychiatry," *The Journal of the History of Medicine and Allied Sciences* 61 (January 2006) 1–25. Subsequent to that article, the critique of the pendulum metaphor has been elaborated in Nicolas Rasmussen, *On Speed: The Many Lives of Amphetamine* (New York: New York University Press, 2008) and Martyn

Pickersgill, "From Psyche to Soma? Changing Accounts of Antisocial Personality Disorders in the *American Journal of Psychiatry,*" *History of Psychiatry* 21, 3 (2010) 294–311.

7 On the difference between living and dead metaphors, see Paul Ricoeur, *Time and Narrative* (Kathleen McLaughlin and David Pellauer, trans., Chicago: University of Chicago Press, 1984), ix: "The metaphor is alive as long as we can perceive, through the new semantic pertinence . . . the resistance of the words in their ordinary sense and therefore their incompatibility at the level of a literal interpretation of the sentence." On historical metaphors, see also Robert Nisbet, *Social Change and History: Aspects of the Western Theory of Development* (London: Oxford University Press, 1969).

8 Nathan Hale, *Freud and the Americans: The Beginnings of Psychoanalysis in the United States, 1876–1917* (New York: Oxford University Press, 1971), 50.

9 For an introduction to the historiographical issues raised by this tension, see Andrew Scull, "Somatic Treatments and the Historiography of Psychiatry," *History of Psychiatry* V (1994) 1–12; H. Mersky, "Somatic Treatments, Ignorance, and the Historiography of Psychiatry," *History of Psychiatry* V (1994) 387–391; Andrew Scull, "Psychiatrists and Historical 'Facts,' Part One: The Historiography of Somatic Treatments," *History of Psychiatry* VI (1995) 225–241.

10 Roy R. Grinker and Helen V. McLean, "The Course of a Depression Treated by Psychotherapy and Metrazol," *Psychosomatic Medicine* 2, 2 (April 1940) 119–138.

11 Norman Levy and Roy Grinker, "Psychological Observations in Affective Psychoses Treated with Combined Convulsive Shock and Psychotherapy," *The Journal of Nervous and Mental Disease* 97, 6 (June 1943) 623.

12 Harry Stack Sullivan, *Conceptions of Modern Psychiatry* (Washington, D.C.: The William Alanson White Psychiatric Foundation, 1947), 73.

13 Cited as a personal communication in L. Bryce Boyer, "Fantasies Concerning Convulsive Therapy," *Psychoanalytic Review* 39 (1952) 252–270. Boyer was a psychoanalyst who championed the idea that countertransference could be used positively in therapeutic settings. He also advocated the use of psychoanalytic techniques for severe mental illness, and not simply for mild neurosis. Wolfgang Saxon, "L. Bryce Boyer," *New York Times,* August 26, 2000.

14 T. M. Luhrmann, *Of Two Minds: The Growing Disorder in American Psychiatry* (New York: Alfred A. Knopf, 2000).

15 Bryce Boyer used the quote as an example of a vitriolic and irrational response to somatic therapy in his "Fantasies Concerning Convulsive Therapy." The quote is used as a prime exhibit of psychoanalytic hostility to ECT in Shorter, *A History of Psychiatry,* 222.

16 Shorter, *History of Psychiatry,* 222.

17 Frank Sulloway has thoroughly discussed what he calls Freud's "cryptobiologism," in *Freud: Biologist of the Mind* (New York: Basic Books, 1979).

18 Sigmund Freud, "Psychoanalysis and the War Neuroses," in James Strachey, trans., *The Standard Edition of the Complete Psychological Works of Sigmund Freud* (London: Hogarth Press, 1953–1974), 211–215. Psychoanalytic authors who wrote about ECT did not cite Freud's discussion of electrical therapies. This may reflect their recognition that convulsive therapy had a different clinical rationale, but in some cases, their interpretation of ECT's efficacy was similar to Freud's understanding of non-convulsive electrical treatment.

19 Freud, "Psychoanalysis and the War Neuroses."

20 Freud doubted that the same level of cruelty was evident in Austria.

21 On non-convulsive use of electrical stimulation in military psychiatry, see Ben Shephard, *A War of Nerves: Soldiers and Psychiatrists in the Twentieth Century* (Cambridge: Harvard University Press, 2001), 12, 76, 100–103.

22 One sign of this conflation may be in Shephard's index, which lists all psychiatric uses of electricity under the heading "Electric Shock Treatment," and does not differentiate convulsive therapy—although the text of the book does. See Shepard, *A War of Nerves,* 206 and 477.

23 Joseph Berke, *I Haven't Had to Go Mad Here* (Harmondsworth: Penguin Books, 1979, originally published as *Butterfly Man,* 1977), 71–72. Elaine Showalter cited Berke's interpretation as an explanation for the success of Sylvia Plath's ECT. Writing in 1985, during the dawn of the resurgence of biological psychiatry, Showalter assumed that if ECT worked, it would be due to a psychological process, not a physiological one. Showalter, *The Female Malady,* 217.

24 Pressman, *Last Resort,* 83–84.

25 See Otto Fenichel, *The Psychoanalytic Theory of Neurosis* (New York: W. W. Norton, 1945), 569.

26 Braslow, *Mental Ills and Bodily Cures,* 96.

27 Valenstein, *Great and Desperate Cures,* 180–184.

28 Gregory Zilboorg, "The Fundamental Conflict with Psychoanalysis," *International Journal of Psychoanalysis* 20 (1939) 480–492. This article was cited by Boyer as an example of analytic prejudice opposed to ECT, but Zilboorg does not mention ECT in the article, only chemically induced convulsion therapies.

29 Braslow, *Mental Ills and Bodily Cures,* 100.

30 Edith Vowinckel Weigert, "Psychoanalytical Notes on Sleep and Convulsion Treatment in Functional Psychoses," *Psychiatry* 3 (1940) 189–209. Like many of the psychiatrists discussed here, both analysts and "somaticists," Weigert was an immigrant who left Europe during the rise of fascism in Germany and Italy. She settled and practiced in the Baltimore area. Her article on chemical convulsive therapy was cited by several later psychoanalytic authors on related somatic treatments.

31 Weigert, "Psychoanalytical Notes," 189.

32 Eric P. Mosse, "Electroshock and Personality Structure," *Journal of Nervous and Mental Diseases* 104 (July 1946) 296–302. Mosse was born and educated in Germany, came to the United States in 1933, and was the author of a book about psychiatry for the lay public, *The Conquest of Loneliness* (New York: Random House, 1957).

33 John A. P. Millet and Eric P. Mosse, "On Certain Psychological Aspects of Electroshock Therapy," *Psychosomatic Medicine* 6, 3 (1944) 226–236. See especially 232–232.

34 Mosse, "Electroshock and Personality Structure," 297.

35 Mosse, "Electroshock and Personality Structure," 298.

36 Mosse, "Electroshock and Personality Structure," 298, emphasis in original.

37 Mosse, "Electroshock and Personality Structure," 298.

38 Mosse, "Electroshock and Personality Structure," 300.

39 Commentary by Dr. Foster Kennedy, *Journal of Nervous and Mental Diseases* 104 (July 1946) 320. Kennedy wrote that Mosse has "made an effort to combine, willy-nilly, something with which we have been familiar during the last 30 years in psychological mechanism as described by Freud, with an entirely new instrument of treatment, and tried to belittle the latter in terms of the former." Kennedy had been using ECT almost daily since 1940, and asserted confidently that the death threat played no part in the cure of his patients.

40 Millet and Mosse, "On Certain Psychological Aspects of Electroshock Therapy," 231.

41 Millet and Mosse, "On Certain Psychological Aspects of Electroshock Therapy," 231.

42 Ben H. Gottesfeld and Calvin Barker, "An Interpretive Study of Subjective Response to Electric Shock Therapy," *Digest of Neurology and Psychiatry* 14, 642 (1946) 642–648.

43 Sylvia Plath, *The Bell Jar* (New York: Bantam Books, 1971, originally published 1963), 118.

44 Shorter claims, as evidence, that the Group for the Advancement of Psychiatry— a psychiatric organization associated with the Menninger Clinic—first opposed ECT "while not condemning it outright," and later "backtracked" to oppose only its "indiscriminate" use. Shorter, *A History of Psychiatry*, 222. In fact, the group's first statement on the subject opposes only indiscriminate use, and this statement condemns both extravagant claims made on ECT's behalf, as well as uninformed denunciation of ECT from other quarters; Group for the Advancement of Psychiatry, *Shock Therapy*, report no. 1, September 15, 1947.

45 Perry, *Psychiatrist of America*, 197. It is also not clear that Sullivan should really be considered an analyst. Although he was sympathetic to many psychoanalytic tenets (as many psychiatrists of the time were), and underwent a psychoanalysis, Sullivan was very critical of aspects of psychoanalysis; see Perry, 259. According to Perry, Sullivan only called himself as a psychoanalyst "after politics with words had become a big and dangerous game in psychoanalytic/psychiatric circles, particularly along the eastern seaboard." Perry, 362–363.

46 Charles H. Kellner, John T. Pritchett, Mark D. Beale, and Edward C. Coffey, *Handbook of ECT* (Washington, D.C.: American Psychiatric Press, 1997), 3.

47 Kalinowsky and Hoch, *Shock Treatments and Other Somatic Procedures in Psychiatry.*

48 Kalinowsky and Hoch, *Shock Treatments*, v.

49 Kalinowsky and Hoch, *Shock Treatments*, 237–240.

50 Kalinowsky and Hoch, *Shock Treatments*, 241–242.

51 Sydney Pulver, "Regulation of Electroconvulsive Therapy," *Michigan Law Review* 75 (1976–1977) 363–412.

52 In Kellner et al., *Handbook of ECT*, the authors mark the turning point as the "classic research" by J.O. Ottoson in the early 1960s that established that the convulsion was crucial to efficacy. See J.O. Ottoson, "Experimental Studies of the Mode of Action of Electroconvulsive Therapy," *Acta Psychiatrica Neurologica Scandinavia Supplement* 145 (1960) 1–141 and J.O. Ottoson, "Seizure Characteristics and Therapeutic Efficiency in Electroconvulsive Therapy: An Analysis of the Antidepressive Efficiency of Grand Mal and Lidocaine-Modified Seizures," *Journal of Nervous and Mental Diseases* 135 (1962) 239–251. But Kalinowsky and Hoch had already proposed that convulsions were necessary for therapeutic effect; see *Shock Treatments*, 238–239.

53 See UK ECT Review Group, "Efficacy and Safety of Electroconvulsive Therapy."

54 Healy, *The Creation of Psychopharmacology*, 343.

55 Millet and Mosse, "On Certain Psychological Aspects of Electroshock Therapy," 227.

56 Metzl, *Prozac on the Couch*. Metzl's account is compelling in many respects, but is weakened by a tendency to treat any sexist practices and assumptions as "psychoanalytic" rather than showing how they are sexist in specifically psychoanalytic ways; while there is no doubt a rich history of sexism within psychoanalysis, sexism is far too diverse in its origins, and psychoanalysis too diverse in its manifestations, for the two to be so strongly equated.

57 For example, Pressman relates that Roy Grinker criticized proponents of lobotomy in the early 1940s, charging them with an agenda of hoping to swing the therapeutic pendulum from psychological to somatic methods. Pressman, *Last Resort*, 132.

5 "Total Rejection of Psychiatry"

ECT and the Antipsychiatry Movement

In "Howl," with its bitter references to futile somatic psychiatric treatments including ECT, Allen Ginsberg was addressing his friend Carl Solomon, whom he met while both were patients at the Greystone Park Psychiatric Hospital in New Jersey. The circumstances behind their admissions were rather different. Ginsberg's followed his arrest after stolen goods were found in his apartment and a vehicle he was riding in. Solomon's admission was voluntary. His "Report from the Asylum" provided an account of insulin coma therapy that was both vivid and dismal.[1] Solomon began the essay by citing Kalinowsky and Hoch's textbook, which he rightly named as the era's definitive work. He cited it to show, as the authors conceded, that the reason ECT worked was mysterious. Solomon wrote:

> This confession of ignorance (and it is extended to both insulin and electric shock therapies), by two of the men who usually place the electrodes on the heads of mental patients at one of four psychiatric hospitals, certainly opens the field of inquiry to the sensitive layman as well as to the technician.[2]

But the mystery of the efficacy of shock treatments would prove to be a minor complaint. Solomon conceded the fact of his illness early in "Report from the Asylum," but concluded the essay with what he called a "total rejection" of psychiatry, and indeed by questioning the category of madness itself. He quoted French poet Antonin Artaud, whose involuntary ECT itself became notorious: "A vicious society has invented psychiatry to defend itself from the investigations of certain superior lucid minds whose intuitive powers were disturbing to it."[3]

Beat literature was an opening salvo in the attacks on psychiatry that would collectively be called the antipsychiatry movement. Another example is Seymour Krim, whose brother had a lobotomy—which Seymour cosigned for—that ended in death by cerebral hemorrhage.[4] When Seymour himself was 33 and living in Greenwich Village, he wrote, "The pressures in my head exploded." He ran barefoot in the street, spat at family members, exposed himself in public, and ultimately was taken to a private institution in Westchester, where he received insulin coma therapy.[5] He complained there that the causes of his illness were never explored, and he was treated condescendingly, like a child. After discharge, he moved back to Manhattan, where he stayed at a cheap Broadway hotel because he felt too ashamed to go back to the Village. After a suicide attempt he was again institutionalized, and received ECT at a Long Island hospital. Here again, he complained that most of the patients in the hospital were not truly insane, but simply people with problems, and that there was no serious attempt to make them independent adults, but only efforts to suppress their problems with pills and shock treatments. A mental hospital, he said, "is not an asylum or a sanctuary in the old-fashioned sense: it is just a roped-off side-street of modern existence, rife with as many contradictions, half-truths and lousy architecture as life itself."[6] His psychiatrist, by contrast, touted the values of adjustment to society and called Greenwich Village a "psychotic community."[7] Krim regarded his cure more of a chastisement than a true healing process, and he considered it necessary to completely rethink the idea of insanity. The best minds of his generation, he concluded, were destroyed not by madness, but by a certain interpretation of madness.[8]

Historian Gerald Grob has argued that it was the influence of the Freudian domination of psychiatric thought, and the expansion of that way of thinking into everyday life, that above all led to the antipsychiatry movement.[9] Freudian psychiatry, he argues, encouraged a social activist psychiatry. By moving attention away from biology and to the social environment, it led psychiatry to aspire to leading social reform, assuming a priest-like mantle. This overreach, Grob maintained, led to the reaction of antipsychiatry.

Grob has the wrong emphasis. It is true that over the first half of the twentieth century, psychiatrists insisted on their relevance to wider social problems, as opposed to restricting their attention to the severely ill. And psychoanalysis did play a major role in this—not surprisingly, as Freud hoped his ideas about psychopathology would yield a gain for normal psychology. Psychiatry's colonization of everyday life had its critics, such as Philip Rieff in *The Triumph of the Therapeutic*.[10] But it was primarily institutional and biological psychiatry that outraged psychiatry's critics in the 1960s. The people Grob names as the leaders of antipsychiatry, such as Szasz and Laing, who were clear that their main targets were involuntary hospitalizations, involuntary treatments, and somatic treatments, particularly shock treatments. I see little reason not to take them at their word. Szasz and Laing both were trained as psychoanalysts, and while they were hardly practitioners of any remotely orthodox psychoanalysis, neither did they repudiate the psychoanalytic approach. Szasz made a point of excluding psychoanalysis from his critique of psychiatry, on the grounds that psychoanalysis was a voluntary contractual relationship and therefore not a deprivation of liberty.[11] But there is more at stake here than my disagreement with another historian. As Michael Staub has recently argued, the antipsychiatry movement has received a great deal of scorn since the waning of its influence.[12] Just as discarded clinical practices and theories deserve recovery from the enormous condescension of posterity, so too do the reactions, and overreactions, to them. There were excesses to the antipsychiatry movement. But its proponents were responding to real problems in somatic psychiatry, had important insights, and in ironic ways may have contributed to the progress of the kinds of psychiatry they abhorred.

There were other seeds of the antipsychiatry movement that were planted before the treatises of its major avatars: physicians such as Szasz and Laing, and sociologists like Goffman, and Thomas Scheff, who developed the labeling theory of mental illness, positing a wholly social etiological theory.[13] Novels such as *Snake Pit,* as well as investigative reporting on conditions in mental hospitals, established the critique of psychiatry, especially involuntary psychiatry, as a genre of writing. The antipsychiatry movement was born out of the experience of the mental hospitals. We have seen that there were indeed punitive uses of ECT in the hospitals, and moreover that the line between the coercive and the therapeutic was not always so easy to draw neatly. From this it was perhaps a short step to begin wondering whether enforcing conformity was in fact psychiatry's principal function, and not an unfortunate or occasional by-product. It was, of course, a step made easier by the wider questioning of authority that the long 1960s became known for. When that questioning took the form of wondering if it was in fact society that was insane, the very category of insanity as an illness would be questioned too.

As such an environment developed in the late 1950s and early 1960s, ECT posed a problem. ECT is justified only on the grounds that it is an effective treatment for severe mental illness. If the so-called illnesses it treats are not illnesses at all, ECT cannot be seen as therapeutic in any sense. While Prozac and other psychiatric medications have occasionally had boosters so enthusiastic that they have been recommended for purposes of "cosmetic psychopharmacology," or enhancement to make one "better than well," no proponent of ECT has ever suggested it should be used in healthy people.

This chapter focuses on the role and representation of ECT in antipsychiatry. I do not aim to provide a full history of the antipsychiatry and radical psychiatry movements. These movements have not received enough attention from historians, who have often adopted the paradigms of the movement more than they have historicized it. This situation is beginning to change. An important point that has been emphasized in new work on the subject, such as Michael Staub's, is that the intellectual leaders of these movements did not hold identical views.[14] There were, though, certain core ideas that became widespread, and remain influential among some critics of psychiatry. These were 1) that madness was—or could be—a form of protest against social norms, 2) that psychiatry was a form of social control in the guise of medical treatment, 3) that the regimens of drugs and other somatic treatments punished deviance, 4) that asylums were essentially detention camps for social undesirables, and 5) that mental illness was a construct with no basis in science.[15] It is easy to see that ECT would be controversial at best among people who were adopting these as premises.

Although there were antecedents, Thomas Szasz's 1961 *The Myth of Mental Illness* was a forceful opening round of the antipsychiatry movement.[16] It was the first of a series of books in which Szasz would, over the course of a long career, develop one of the most influential critiques of psychiatry. Born in Hungary, Szasz was a fully trained psychiatrist, as well as a psychoanalyst, who was professor of psychiatry at the State University of New York Upstate Medical University. He was a committed libertarian, and his critique of psychiatry was embedded in broader advocacy for personal freedom. The core idea in his criticism of psychiatry was that so-called mental illnesses should not be in the purview of medicine at all. So-called mental illnesses, he maintained, were simply problems in living, and in most cases, problems for *other people,* such as family members, not for the allegedly ill person. He did, though, argue that individuals might self-label as mentally ill to exploit the bogus category of mental illness in order to get access to the benefits of the sick role. He consistently insisted that illness could never be properly diagnosed solely on the basis of behavior or mood, but only when medicine could identify visible lesions. Thus, Alzheimer's disease, although it could only be diagnosed in a living person on the basis of behavior, could qualify as a bona fide illness because medical research had identified visible brain abnormalities in the bodies of Alzheimer's sufferers once deceased.

One of the greatest weaknesses of his thought was a failure to provide adequate justification for this criterion of illness. There was, after all, a time before Alzheimer, when brain abnormalities had not been identified in anyone with dementia; were the sufferers not legitimately sick then? If we were to find brain abnormalities in someone with, say, social anxiety disorder, would we then have to move it from the column of myth to the column of illness?

Szasz did not extend his criticism to voluntary psychotherapy or psychoanalysis, which, as noted earlier, he regarded as contractual relations entered into willingly, and therefore not a limitation on the personal freedom he cherished. What he did object to were involuntary hospitalization, and involuntary treatments.[17] At times, Szasz actually *equated* psychiatry with involuntary treatments, which amounted to semantic legerdemain—it is of course a lot easier to mount a critique of psychiatry if your definition of psychiatry excludes all voluntary treatments.

Szasz said surprisingly little about ECT in his earlier works. Perhaps he thought that, if you accept the premise that mental illness is not a real thing, the barbarity of ECT is self-evident. Szasz's early work was devoted to establishing that premise. ECT is not mentioned in *The Myth of Mental Illness*. It appears briefly in his 1970 work *The Manufacture of Madness: A Comparative Study of the Inquisition and the Mental Health Movement.*[18] There, he quoted Cerletti as saying to a colleague after the first use of ECT on a human, "When I saw the patient's reaction, I thought to myself: this ought to be abolished."[19] I have not seen this comment mentioned in eyewitness accounts of the first ECT. Whether Cerletti said this at the time or not, though, it is misleading to sum up his attitude with this quote, as Cerletti was proud of his invention, and promoted its use.

Szasz wrote a full-blown critique of ECT late in his life in a chapter of *Coercion as Cure,* one of his last books. The title of the chapter, "Iatrogenic Epilepsy," is itself an argument. Iatrogenic disease is disease induced by medical treatment. ECT operates by inducing seizures, which is a symptom of a real disease, epilepsy, and Szasz expected us to be outraged by this. Szasz put great stock in precedents from other (he would have said "real") areas of medicine, but it is common practice in medicine to perform procedures— surgery, and chemotherapy for cancer, for example—that cause unhealthful effects in healthy people. Szasz noted that the original clinical rationale for ECT—the supposed inverse relationship between schizophrenia and epilepsy—is dubious now. He went on, as most writers hostile to ECT do, to detail the story of the first ECT treatment in Italy, which was performed involuntarily, and continued even after the patient protested. But then Szasz also cited the evidence from subsequent ECT patients of the benefits they have gotten from the treatment. Szasz mentioned well-known ECT patients, including Dick Cavett and Sherwin Nuland, who have spoken eloquently about the relief ECT brought them. But having cited them, Szasz did not consider the obvious challenge they pose to his argument, not even to refute the challenge.[20]

Szasz's influence must be given its due. Involuntary psychiatric incarcerations and treatments do raise significant ethical issues that were inadequately addressed before his work appeared. He does not deserve sole credit for raising them, but he certainly injected into public debate a radical form of questioning of psychiatric practice. Szasz was influential, but was not always happy about how his ideas were adopted. He was popular in the amorphous movement called the "counter-culture" in the 1960s, but felt little affinity with it. He also has been "credited' with contributing intellectual support to the de-institutionalization movement, but that movement rarely questioned that there was such a thing as mental illness that needed to be treated, instead emphasizing that patients could be better served outside of institutions.

Szasz is conventionally regarded as part of the antipsychiatry movement, but just as he disavowed the views of many of his followers, he disavowed the label antipsychiatry. He saw antipsychiatry, which he identified with psychiatrists R.D. Laing and David Cooper, as merely a branch of psychiatry, and one which had no more basis in science than mainstream psychiatry (perhaps even less), and was no less threatening to personal freedom.

There is one very concrete measure of the difference between Szasz and some of the other canonical figures of antipsychiatry: most of the others did not question the reality of mental illness, even if they made radical criticisms of the ways it was treated or of prevailing conceptions of its cause. Goffman is a good illustration, because Goffman was one who was very influenced by Szasz's program.[21] Despite that, Goffman's own work on asylums did not question whether the inmates were truly ill. He was more interested in understanding the social dynamics within the asylum as he built his wider critique of what he called total institutions. ECT played a role as a disciplinary tool, but not because the inmates were, as Szasz would have it, not really ill, but more because it was the nature of these institutions to enforce strict discipline. Scheff's labeling theory fell in a tradition of sociological critique of the origins and consequences of deviancy in general. It was a theory of the origins of mental illness, not a questioning of its reality. Scheff proposed that everyone engages in deviance to some extent, and that when other social actors called it "madness," one would internalize the label and become truly unwell.

By arguing that social life itself presented all of us with "crazy" contradictions, Laing's thought might seem to suggest continuity between sanity and insanity. His argument was an extension, in some ways, of the problem Frantz Fanon posed from his experience as a psychiatrist in Algeria during its war for independence: what was the point of trying to make people mentally healthy during the manifestly unhealthy condition of a an anti-colonial war?[22] Laing developed this line of thought by extending the idea of a manifestly unhealthy society, even apart from the extreme conditions of an anti-colonial war. Laing also avoided the clinical language of psychiatry in interactions with patients, because he thought that language erected a barrier between him and them. But while he saw his patients' problems as problems of adaptation, as understandable response to social reality, there is no question that he thought that they were, in fact, in need of some kind of clinical care. In this respect, Szasz was quite justified in distancing himself.

But where Szasz and Laing were united was in their special distaste for somatic interventions. For Laing, this distaste grew out of his early training as a psychiatrist in the 1950s. He recoiled from the use of lobotomy, insulin coma, and ECT.[23] "I was beginning to suspect," Laing said, "that insulin and electric shocks, not to mention lobotomy and the whole environment of a psychiatric unit, were ways of destroying people and driving them mad."[24] Laing developed his own inpatient treatment center in London, which would have many unorthodox features but would not use any shock treatments or lobotomy. Patients were drawn to it, and Laing kept a trunk full of the letters from people asking to be admitted.[25]

Mary Barnes was probably the most famous patient to be treated in Laing's clinic. Barnes co-wrote her story with Laingian psychiatrist Joseph Berke, and it was adapted into a Broadway play.[26] Barnes referred to ECT as the "so-called treatment" she received at a conventional mental hospital after a breakdown in 1952, and lamented that at the time she was unaware that it was, as she came to think, a punitive one.[27] Berke saw the mental hospital as an extension of the oppressive world of the family, but with more developed tools for discipline, such as tranquilizers and electric shock.[28]

These are contrasted with the warmth and humanity Barnes felt from Laing and other clinicians who helped her explore the meaning of her suffering through artistic expression. Laing appears in the story as a figure akin to *Snake Pit*'s Dr. Kik, a talk therapist exploring meaning rather than suppressing symptoms.

Laing tends to be remembered as a radical, for his critique of social context, and for his apparent questioning of the border between madness and sanity. On the latter point, he insisted that he was misunderstood, that he wished to understand madness in the context of the social order, but recognized that it was not a healthy adaptation to it. Laing's departure from the psychiatric mainstream was indeed dramatic, and he adopted some techniques that seem kooky in retrospect.[29] But his clinical approach was rooted in an old and hardy psychiatric tradition that has held that, for all their suffering and real difference from the sane, the mad are people who can be reached and understood if treated as people. This way of thinking has been expressed by figures as diverse as Dorothea Dix, Sigmund Freud, and Harry Stack Sullivan. For none of these was this stance a rejection of the idea of mental illness, or of the idea that the mad needed treatment. Laing always wanted treatment for patients, just not somatic treatments. To the end of his career, he not only shunned ECT in treatment, but preferred to work with patients who had not received it from others.[30] This was consistent with his belief that symptoms were vivid signs pointing to the meaning of the patient's pain, although signs whose tangled appearance made them challenging to decode. For Laing, ECT's effectiveness at relieving symptoms was one of its flaws. With the symptoms unavailable, a route to the origin of the suffering, and the hope of a deeper transformation, were blocked.

Antipsychiatry is usually discussed with reference to its intellectual leaders. But it was also a social movement with broad influence on popular thought. This should not be exaggerated. Throughout the 1960s and early 1970s, Americans mostly continued to believe in mental illness, and to use psychiatric services. Popular faith in psychiatry may have actually increased during this period. Nevertheless, antipsychiatry put down deep roots.[31] The notion that people in the asylum might in fact be the sane ones, expressed, for example, in the popular movie *King of Hearts* (1966), became a staple of lay thought. A glimpse into this can be seen in Mark Vonnegut's memoir *Eden Express*.[32] Vonnegut, son of the novelist Kurt, was a young man in the 1960s, who believed with all his friends that Szasz was right, that mental illness was a myth, until he had a psychotic breakdown himself. The book concludes with his insistence on the reality of mental illness and the need for psychiatric treatment when it is present, a view he has also advocated in another more recent memoir.[33]

But what we might call "lay antipsychiatry" also took other forms, which did not necessarily involve questioning the reality of mental illness or the need for some kind of treatment. One other form of it was the psychiatric survivor movements and literature, which often expressed a wish for psychotherapy of some kind, but lambasted involuntary treatments and somatic treatments.

The *Madness Network News* was a psychiatric survivors' magazine of the early 1970s that illustrates this posture, and its contents included some bitter testimony regarding ECT.[34] That contributors drew on the intellectual resources of the antipsychiatry movement is evident in their rejection of the term "patient," and in the particular animus against somatic treatments: "If you thought you were going crazy, and if you wound up with 'professional help,' you may have seen how frequently that 'help' is delivered through a syringe or a pill."[35] One contributor wrote, based on her experience in a mental hospital, that simply crying could get you labeled depressed, in which case you could get ECT, and quoted Kesey to the effect that no one ever wants a second shock treatment.[36] Another contributor conceded that in mental hospitals many patients went for ECT eagerly, but that others did so very apprehensively, and complained of side effects including "headache, confusion, exhaustion, and permanent memory loss."[37] This contributor also claimed that many patients concealed their fear of the treatment for fear of being considered paranoid, and thus a better fit for the treatment. One particularly resentful account complained of serious cognitive losses, and compared ECT doctors to war criminals or Nazi doctors.

One influential example of survivor literature was Leonard Roy Frank's *The History of Shock Treatment,* an anthology of writings on ECT. Frank, one of the editors of the *Madness Network News Reader,* dedicated his book "to all those engaged in the struggle against psychiatric tyranny."[38] Frank had been an involuntary psychiatric inmate for eight months in 1962–1963. His diagnosis was "paranoid schizophrenia," and he was "forcibly subjected to a course of combined insulin coma-convulsive treatment (50 insulin coma and 35 electroconvulsive treatments) at Twin Pines Hospital in Belmont, California, a peninsula suburb of San Francisco. The procedure resulted in a total and permanent amnesia for the two-year period preceding the last shock treatment."[39] In 1964, Frank discovered Szasz's work, and came to know Szasz personally.[40] Frank did not advocate banning ECT, but argued that it should always be voluntary.

For his anthology, Frank scoured the literature on ECT. He relied more on professional testimony than that of survivors. Frank cited numerous psychiatrists who claimed that ECT works by causing brain damage, or who thought the erasure of memory was the reason for therapeutic benefit. It is more than a little one-sided. Very few of the many professional reports that disputed brain damage, or which judged permanent memory loss to be rare, are included. His collection represents the case against the treatment in distilled form. He provided the voices of patients, but for the most part only the voices of patients who shared his negative experience. That said, the history he provides is no more selective than some accounts that emphasize only ECT's therapeutic benefits.

Being Sane in Insane Places

One account of the origin of ECT tells the story this way:

> Here's how it came about: two psychiatrists were visiting a slaughter-house, for God knows what perverse reason, and were watching cattle being killed by a blow between the eyes with a sledgehammer. They noticed that not all the cattle were killed, that some would fall to the floor in a state that greatly resembled epileptic convulsion. 'Ah, zo,' the first doctor says. 'Zis is exactly vot ve need for our patients—zee induced *fit!*' His colleague agreed, of course. It was known that men coming out of an epileptic convulsion were inclined to be calmer and more peaceful for a time, and that violent cases completely out of contact were able to carry on rational conversations after a convulsion. No one knew why; they still don't. But it was obvious that if a seizure could be induced in non-epileptics, great benefits might result. And here, before them, stood a man inducing seizures every so often with remarkable aplomb.[41]

This passage is from *Cuckoo's Nest;* it is the words of the patient Harding, explaining to protagonist Randall McMurphy what is in store for him if he challenges the authority of Nurse Ratched.

If *The Myth of Mental Illness* was the emblematic treatise of the revolt against psychiatry, its close contemporary *One Flew Over the Cuckoo's Nest* was its prime fictional representative. *Cuckoo's Nest* is also most likely the strongest cultural association most people have with ECT. For many prospective patients Forman's film adaptation is the first thing that comes to mind when ECT is mentioned, although that effect may be waning for younger patients. ECT actually takes place in a very limited portion of both the novel and the film. But it haunts the entire story as an ominous threat.

Note, though, that even in *Cuckoo's Nest,* ECT actually does McMurphy very little harm. It is a source of terror for his fellow patient Cheswick, especially in the film, but McMurphy emerges from it if anything revital-ized. McMurphy appears in the end as a "vegetable," but this is due to his lobotomy, not ECT.[42]

Psychiatrists who use ECT will often complain about the way *Cuckoo's Nest* sensationalized ECT. The action is lurid in some respects, but the depiction of ECT in the story is realistic in some ways, too, for the time the story takes place. Clinicians recognized that the treatment was frighten-ing. Harding gives several descriptions of ECT in the novel, none of which are fanciful. This quote may be particularly surprising to those who view *Cuckoo's Nest* as an unambiguous vilification of ECT:

> [ECT] isn't always used for punitive measures, as our nurse uses it, and it isn't pure sadism on the staff's part, either. A number of supposed irre-coverables were brought back into contact with shock, just as a number

were helped with lobotomy and leucotomy. Shock treatment has some advantages; it's cheap, quick, and entirely painless. It simply induces a seizure.[43]

The story of *Cuckoo's Nest* reverses the more typical gender dynamic of ECT. In reality it was overwhelmingly administered by male clinicians and the patients have probably been mostly women. Arguably, *Cuckoo's Nest* is less about madness and psychiatry than it is a story of women who prevent men from being men, and the terrible, castrating fate that comes to one man who challenges this and tries to restore virility to the men.[44] In this sense, despite its self-congratulatory celebration of non-conformity, *Cuckoo's Nest* is a very conventional story.

One question McMurphy's story explores—what happens to sane people in insane places—was an old one well before Kesey's time. Andrew Scull has recently showed that Victorian fiction was replete with stories of sane people in insane asylums, sometimes just trapped there as sane, sometimes contaminated into madness.[45] It was a theme also echoed in the 1963 American movie *Shock Corridor,* about an undercover reporter who goes into a mental hospital to investigate a murder and receives shock treatments. He is left with a damaged mind, and indefinitely institutionalized. Two years before the film version of *Cuckoo's Nest* was released, this theme would receive classic social science expression in D. L. Rosenhan's paper "On Being Sane in Insane Places," an account of the experience of sociologists who checked themselves into a mental hospital to see if clinicians could tell the difference. In Rosenhan's telling, the clinicians did have some trouble with this, although the "real" patients did not.[46]

The Twilight and Legacy of Antipsychiatry

Kesey's book appeared during the first stirrings of the antipsychiatry movement, while Forman's film came around the end of it. The film left the public with searing images of involuntary treatments. But by the time it appeared, in 1975, assertions that mental illness was a myth had already seen their days of greatest influence. The revisions to the Diagnostic and Statistical Manual of Mental Disorders would culminate in a third edition that would be a most emphatic assertion of biological psychiatry. The era of DSM-III and subsequent editions have certainly been times of a lot of debate about disease mongering, the ever-widening range of behaviors that would be seen as mental illness, and the role of pharmaceutical companies in promoting diseases. Some of the intellectual repertoire of the antipsychiatry movement has been adopted in these debates. But the basic existence of severe mental illness has been less often questioned, and the rooting of that illness in biology, or chemistry, or the brain, or whatever one considers the basic materiality of the self, has had a broad, although not unquestioned, hegemony.

The antipsychiatry movement was motivated by real problems, both the-oretical and practical, in psychiatry and in society. To reduce it to an irratio-nal prejudice is to idealize medical and psychiatric science. And, in the end, the downfall of antipsychiatry was due less to science than to patient expe-rience and concerns. The most powerful arguments against antipsychiatry are not found in any clinical trial or brain imaging. Clinical trials and brain imaging, on the contrary, can only acquire power if backed by cultural force to deem a condition an illness. It really does not matter what doctors think the success rate of a treatment for a disease is if laypeople are not prepared to think it is a disease. Nor does it matter if you can show differences in the brains of diagnosed people from people without a diagnosis if there is no cultural force behind the seeing the diagnosis as valid. Imagine if one could show a difference in the brains of people who like to eat meat and those of people who prefer vegetarianism. Would this be grounds for considering one of the preferences a disease—and if so, which one? The most powerful arguments against antipsychiatry are not scientific, but are in cultural docu-ments such as Mark Vonnegut's *Eden Express,* the moving memoir of a man who himself rejected mental illness as a "myth," until he had one.

By most accounts, ECT use decreased in the 1960s and early 1970s. I do not believe this has been documented definitively, but it certainly is the uniform impression of clinicians who lived through the period.[47] The anti-psychiatry movement probably contributed to that decline. But it should not be exaggerated. For one thing, although the antipsychiatry movement was widespread and influential, the basic counter-tenets—that mental ill-ness is a real thing, and that psychiatry can treat it—remained broadly held. Plus, there were many other factors involved. Most important was the rise of psychopharmacology, when antidepressants and antipsychotics were developed in the 1950s. With both psychiatrists and laypeople already ambivalent about ECT, it is not surprising that some would find hope in the availability of drugs to treat mental illness, and the promise that they would do so more safely than ECT. And both the antipsychiatry movement and the rise of psychopharmacology were among the many reasons for the de-institutionalization movement. Criticism of ECT was thus hitting its harsh-est notes when the procedure itself was becoming increasingly rare for other reasons anyway.

The antipsychiatry movement may have contributed, for a time at least, to a reduction in the use of ECT.[48] But the antipsychiatry movement's oppo-sition to ECT may have, in some ways, actually been a boon to the treat-ment. This may seem unduly contrarian at first glance, but by encouraging the reduction of involuntary treatments, and treatments used for the most coercive purposes, the antipsychiatry made ECT a pill many were more likely to swallow. Without these changes, the revival of ECT might have been far less likely.

The antipsychiatry movement was an attempt to cast ECT (and all of psychiatry) as barbarism. The movement and its leaders have received a fair amount of scorn in recent decades, although there are signs that a more balanced reassessment is underway, just as in the 1990s a more balanced reassessment emerged of the era immediately preceding, the age of shock therapies and lobotomy. Both showed clear excesses in retrospect—in the case of somatic treatments, for example, the zeal of Walter Freeman, and in the case of antipsychiatry, the rejection by Szasz of any therapeutic role for psychiatry whatsoever. But odd as it seems to connect them, both the aggressive somatic treatments of the mid-twentieth century and the antipsychiatry movement were ultimately motivated by the wish to reduce human misery.

Whatever one thinks of the more extreme conclusions of many in the antipsychiatry movement, after decades when psychiatrists produced the frightening treatments insulin coma therapy, Metrazol, lobotomy, and unmodified ECT—all of them administered in many contexts without consent, all with potential for damaging adverse effects—it is not surprising that an antipsychiatry movement would emerge in response. The antipsychiatry movement flourished in a time and context where there were multiple challenges to authority, on many fronts. It was also a time when the cultural authority of the wider field of medicine was facing challenges due to the shocks of the revelations of Nazi medicine, the Tuskegee study, and other ethical abuses. Surely these wider challenges to authority helped inspire antipsychiatry. Just as surely, there were deeply felt and legitimate complaints from survivors of brutal psychiatric treatments.

Antipsychiatry did have a deep and lasting impact. But there were always limits to it. We can see this in the reaction to Thomas Eagleton's nomination for vice president by George McGovern in 1972. When Eagleton's history of depression was revealed—including hospitalization and ECT treatment in the early 1960s—few argued that mental illness was a myth, or a rational response to an insane society. Eagleton's candidacy was quickly regarded as completely unviable. He was dropped from the ticket almost immediately.[49]

ECT survived, or outlasted, the heyday of antipsychiatry. Proponents sometimes view the revival of ECT from the early 1980s as itself a testament to ECT's benefits. The reasoning is that the attachment of such a devastating stigma to a treatment could only have been overcome by the sheer weight of the data. The therapy's manifest benefits in alleviating mental suffering were such that they overwhelmed the public perception of a barbaric treatment. In the minds of the providers, this may in fact have been the case, although they may have found themselves repeatedly recommending it to patients whose dominant image has come from *Cuckoo's Nest*.

But we should also consider some larger contextual factors in the revival of ECT. To begin, the psychiatric profession and the wider culture started to have a greater preoccupation with depression, ECT's primary indication in the 1970s.[50] The 1970s were notable as well for the transition from DSM-II to DSM-III. As many have shown, this was the most significant change in American psychiatric diagnosis, because it marked an intentional downgrading of psychoanalytic perspectives, and was part of a wider shift to what is often called (misleadingly, in my opinion) "biological psychiatry." Both of these developments were signs of the dawning of the age of Prozac. And that age was one where somatic treatments were emphatically welcomed.

A signature text of this new era was Peter Kramer's *Listening to Prozac,* which came out in 1993 and became a bestseller.[51] Many construed this book, wrongly, as a straightforward endorsement of Prozac's benefits.[52] It is in fact an ambivalent book, although the stories Kramer told of patients rapidly feeling "more themselves" or "better than well" probably stoked the demand for antidepressant medication. That Kramer's misgivings about Prozac often went unnoticed was itself a symptom of the culture's growing romance with a biomedical construal of not only mental distress, but of the person, the self. This romance was seen at the highest levels, as President George H. W. Bush pronounced the 1990s to be the "Decade of the Brain."

But Kramer himself observed in *Listening to Prozac* that the romance with the brain and its chemistry was a cultural preoccupation that far outstripped any scientific advances associated with it.[53] This raises a question: why then? Newspaper and magazine articles from the 1990s pronounced Freud dead, on the basis of the apparent efficacy of Prozac. But we had known for many decades prior that somatic treatments could have dramatic effects on the inner life. Malaria fever therapy, insulin coma therapy, lobotomy, Miltown, Thorazine, imipramine, and ECT had already established that by the 1960s. None of them led to widespread collective doubt as to whether social environment, life events, or psychology mattered for the understanding, genesis, and treatment of mental illness (and of course, there was abundant scientific evidence that they did). As Staub has noted, two million people received Thorazine when it first became available in 1954, but biomedical models for the source of mental disorder arguably received less attention, not more, in the years immediately following.[54]

Some authors have associated the new emphasis on the brain with the new economic order ushered in during the 1980s, the set of changes associated with politicians such as Ronald Reagan—the de-emphasis on social welfare, public goods, and social structures.[55] This political and economic culture put renewed emphasis on a hyper-individualistic concept of the person; indeed, Margaret Thatcher famously said that there was no such thing as society. A cultural moment with heightened emphasis on the individual was one that would direct attention to the person's brain chemistry—and also one that would look for the quicker fixes to productivity that Prozac, and ECT, could provide, as compared with dynamic psychotherapy, let alone Freudian psychoanalysis. The age of Prozac, and the revival of ECT, also coincided with the growing popularity in talk therapy of cognitive approaches, as opposed to dynamic approaches. Unlike psychoanalytic psychotherapy, cognitive approaches sought little insight into *why* a depressed person might be having negative thoughts, but rather sought to correct those thoughts, and change behavior. They were also approaches that were hailed by proponents for their speed of action.

All of this may indeed help to explain the revival of ECT. It is a question that deserves more inquiry, although it does not admit of easy empirical demonstration either way. That we were in a new moment, culturally, however, was symbolized by the 1982 publication of Endler's *Holiday of Darkness*. Where the public representations of ECT in the 1960s and 1970s were dominated by negative images, Endler's memoir was the first of a growing number of public testimonies by ECT patients about how they had been helped by the treatment. This does not mean that negative portrayals suddenly stopped appearing. The negative accounts that appeared from 1980 onwards tended to come from people who received involuntary treatment, who felt they were pressured into receiving the treatment, or who felt they received inadequate warning about the risks. And while these did appear, in a growing number of accounts, patients would insist that that ECT was chosen and welcomed. As psychologist and memoirist Martha Manning put it, when an acquaintance asked her how she could let them do this to her, she replied, "I didn't let them do it to me. I asked them to do it."[56]

Manning's account is generally positive toward ECT, although as we will see in the next chapter, she mourned significant memory loss. Endler's memoir is unequivocal. ECT appears in *Holiday of Darkness* as the solution to a deep depression. Part of the power of the book derives from its source—a clinical psychologist who was opposed to the treatment before his personal experience of it. This conversion is common in published ECT memoirs that followed Endler's. Frank Kimball, whose positive account of ECT in the 1940s we looked at in Chapter Two, appears to have gone into the treatment not knowing what to expect. By the 1970s, prospective patients had come to expect the worst. In the decades that followed, several well-known accounts would appear, expressing surprise at ECT's therapeutic effects. Dick Cavett called his ECT treatment "miraculous," "like a magic wand."[57] Other public personalities, such as Kitty Dukakis and Carrie Fisher, would publicize their experience of healing from ECT, and there were memoirs along these lines from less well-known people. Again, all the clinical science in the world would have a certain hollowness if there were not positive patient testimony.

These positive narratives pose an obvious problem for the most vehement critics of ECT practice. It's a problem none of them really address adequately. There continue to be patients whose experience left them hostile to the treatment. Yet among those who had more positive experiences, most wrote accounts that differed from Endler's in an important respect. Rather than being unalloyed celebrations of ECT, most of them contained a bittersweet note. They lamented some loss of memory.

As the revival of ECT proceeded, the therapy remained controversial. But the terms of the controversy shifted. The possibility of adverse cognitive effects such as memory loss, a possibility that had been debated since ECT's inception, became the main source of disagreement. Increasingly, public debate focused less on whether ECT was a punitive or coercive treatment. The questions became instead, what are its costs? And are they worth it?

Notes

1 Carl Solomon, "Report from the Asylum," in Gene Feldman and Max Garten-berg, eds., *The Beat Generation and the Angry Young Men* (New York: The Citadel Press, 1958). Solomon's essay was originally published in 1950, a year after his admission to Greystone.

2 Solomon, "Report from the Asylum," 153–154.

3 Artaud quoted in Solomon, "Report from the Asylum," 162. Artaud was writing about Van Gogh.

4 Seymour Krim, "The Insanity Bit," in Seymour Krim, ed., *The Beats: A Gold Medal Anthology* (Greenwich, CT: Fawcett Publications, Inc., 1960).

5 Krim, "The Insanity Bit," 61–62.

6 Krim, "The Insanity Bit," 66.

7 Krim, "The Insanity Bit," 66–67.

8 Krim, "The Insanity Bit," 68–69.

9 Gerald Grob, "The Attack of Psychiatric Legitimacy in the 1960s: Rhetoric and Reality," *Journal of the History of the Behavioral Sciences* 47, 4 (2011) 398–416.

10 Philip Rieff, *The Triumph of the Therapeutic: Uses of Faith after Freud* (Chicago: University of Chicago Press, 1966).

11 Szasz, *Coercion as Cure.*

12 Staub, *Madness Is Civilization,* 6.

13 See Thomas Scheff, *Being Mentally Ill: A Sociological Theory* (2nd edition, Chicago: Aldine de Gruyter, 1982). In this second edition, Scheff disavowed the strongest theoretical claims he had originally made.

14 This point is made very effectively by Staub, *Madness Is Civilization,* 2.

15 Staub, *Madness Is Civilization,* 3.

16 Thomas Szasz, *The Myth of Mental Illness: Foundations of a Theory of Personal Conduct* (New York: Hoeber-Harper, 1961).

17 See my review of his late book *Coercion as Cure* in *Bulletin of the History of Medicine* 83, 4 (Winter 2009) 797–798.

18 Thomas Szasz, *The Manufacture of Madness: A Comparative Study of the Inquisition and the Mental Health Movement* (New York: Harper Torchbooks, 1970).

19 Szasz, *The Manufacture of Madness,* 31.

20 This paragraph is adapted from my review of *Coercion as Cure,* in the *Bulletin of the History of Medicine* 84, 4 (Winter 2009) 797–798.

21 Staub, *Madness Is Civilization,* 102.

22 Frantz Fanon, *The Wretched of the Earth* (New York: Grove, 1963). Fanon's contributions to anti-colonial thought are well known, but his contributions to antipsychiatric thought may be underestimated. Fanon also witnessed deliberate abuse of ECT as torture, to break people under interrogation. See Frantz Fanon, *A Dying Colonialism* (New York: Grove Press, 1965), 138.

23 John Clay, *R. D. Laing: A Divided Self* (London: Hodder and Stoughton, 1996), 42–43.

24 Quoted in Clay, *R. D. Laing,* 48.

25 Clay, *R. D. Laing,* 131.

26 Mary Barnes and Joseph Berke, "Mary Barnes: Two Accounts of a Journey through Madness," (New York: Harcourt Brace Jovanovich, 1971).

27 Barnes and Berke, "Mary Barnes," 49.

28 Barnes and Berke, "Mary Barnes," 86–87.

29 For example, he facilitated public ritual re-enactments of patients' births.

30 Clay, *R. D. Laing,* 237.

31 The popularization of antipsychiatric thought is demonstrated in Staub, *Madness Is Civilization,* ch. 4.

32 Mark Vonnegut, *The Eden Express* (New York: Bantam Books, 1976).

33 Mark Vonnegut, *Just Like Someone Without a Mental Illness, Only More So* (New York: Delacorte Press, 2010).

34 My discussion of the magazine is based on an anthology of its contents. Sherry Hirsch, Joe Kennedy Adams, Leonard Roy Frank, Wade Hudson, Richard Keene, Gail Krawitz-Keene, David Rochman, and Robert Roth, eds., *Madness Network News Reader* (San Francisco: Glide Publications, 1974).

35 Richard Keene, in the introduction to Hirsch et al., *Madness Network News Reader.*

36 Ann Roy, in Hirsch et al., *Madness Network News Reader,* 23.

37 Joe Kennedy Adams, "You're in for the Shock of Your Life," in Hirsch et al., *Madness Network News Reader,* 82.

38 Leonard Roy Frank, ed., *The History of Shock Treatment* (San Francisco: Leonard Roy Frank, 1978).

39 Frank, *The History of Shock Treatment,* ix.

40 Frank, *The History of Shock Treatment,* x.

41 Ken Kesey, *One Flew Over the Cuckoo's Nest* (New York: The Viking Press, 1962), 163.

42 For Pressman, even this may have represented a defamation of lobotomy. *Last Resort,* 402–403.

43 Kesey, *Cuckoo's Nest,* 163.

44 A number of critics have pointed out the misogyny of *Cuckoo's Nest.* See Stephen L. Tanner, *Ken Kesey* (Boston: Twayne Publishers, 1983), 44–46. Tanner also presents some of the counter-arguments, but they are not very convincing.

45 Andrew Scull, *Madness in Civilization: A Cultural History of Insanity from the Bible to Freud, from the Madhouse to Modern Medicine* (Princeton and Oxford: Princeton University Press, 2015), 239.

46 D.L. Rosenhan, "On Being Sane in Insane Places," *Science* 179, 70 (January 1973) 250–258.

47 See also Staub, *Madness Is Civilization,* 85, on statistics showing the beginning of a reduction in use in the early 1960s.

48 Shorter, *A History of Psychiatry,* 282.

49 Gary Hart, whose own candidacy for president would be rendered unviable by a very different kind of scandal 12 years later, provided an insider's account of the McGovern campaign. When the revelations about Eagleton's illness appeared, McGovern announced that he would stand firmly by the nomination, a decision he would regret because it left no room to maneuver as public opinion asserted itself against Eagleton's place on the ticket. Gary Warren Hart, *Right from the Start: A Chronicle of the McGovern Campaign* (New York: Quadrangle/The New York Times Book Company, 1973), 258.

50 Laura Hirshbein, *American Melancholy* (New Brunswick: Rutgers University Press, 2009).

51 Peter D. Kramer, *Listening to Prozac* (New York: Viking Press, 1993).

52 See, for example, Frederick Crews, "Talking Back to Prozac," *The New York Review of Books,* December 6, 2007. The February 2008 issue of the *New York Review* ran a letter by Kramer complaining that Crews had not read him carefully, that a reading of the book as an advertisement for Prozac missed Kramer's doubts and hesitations. Crews conceded the point in his response.

53 Kramer, *Listening to Prozac.*

54 Staub, *Madness Is Civilization,* 61.

55 See, for example, Andrew Lakoff, *Pharmaceutical Reason: Knowledge and Value in Global Psychiatry* (Cambridge: Cambridge University Press, 2005), and

the editors' introduction to L. Stephen Jacyna and Stephen T. Casper, *The Neurological Patient in History* (Rochester: University of Rochester Press, 2012).

56 Martha Manning, *Undercurrents: A Life beneath the Surface* (New York: HarperSanFrancisco, 1994), 165–166.

57 Jane E. Brody, "Shock Therapy Loses Some of Its Shock Value," *New York Times*, September 19, 2006.

6 The History of a Side Effect
ECT and Memory Loss

"My long-term memory deficits far exceed anything my doctors anticipated, I was advised about, or that are validated by research. . . . How could I be experiencing what I was, if all these experts were saying it wasn't so? I felt that I was being mocked by science."

—Anne Donahue[1]

"Forget the past? We are the past."

—Ellen Wolfe[2]

From the inception of ECT, patients and doctors have expressed concerns about possible cognitive side effects, especially memory loss.[3] Denials that such losses are common are just as old.

Permanent, long-term retrograde memory loss—the loss of already acquired memories—is the most serious possible side effect of modified ECT, but there is controversy about how common it is. Some clinical handbooks describe the risk of this side effect as minimal.[4] Many scientific studies have shown such loss to be possible, but there is no agreement on how common it is. Published narrative accounts of ECT treatment—both positive and negative—refer to major permanent losses in memory more often than they do not. A puzzle is posed: if permanent memory loss from ECT is as rare as many scientific studies claim, why is it so common in narrative accounts? This chapter will examine the history of this side effect by juxtaposing scientific studies and narrative accounts. Just as the history of therapeutics has raised questions about how to regard changing views of efficacy, I raise analogous questions about side effects. Just as efficacy is related to historical context, the meaning and significance of side effects are also historically variable.[5] The idea of a side effect may itself be an unintended side effect of the rise of therapeutic specificity in biomedicine.

Memory loss is a particularly thorny aspect of the ECT debate for several reasons. There is strong scientific consensus that some memory loss of events near in time to the treatment is typical, but that much of the memory, both long-term and short-term, gradually returns for many patients in the following months.[6] There is also agreement that some problems with anterograde memory—the ability to make and keep new memories—may follow the treatment, and this, too, often subsides. *Serious, permanent, long-term amnesia, of events well before the treatment,* is often held to be rare, but I do not believe there is truly a scientific consensus.

There is a lot at stake in this problem. ECT's main indication is severe depression, which is a serious illness, and one that warrants aggressive treatment. Permanent memory loss, though, is a serious side effect, one which might be acceptable to some patients if their illness is painful enough, but one few people would risk lightly. If we are not really sure how great the risk is, the extent of the duty to warn, and the ability to make consent truly informed, are hard to assess.

Clinical claims of negligible risk are distressing for those who do experience severe losses. This has been well expressed by ECT patient Anne Donahue in a memoir of her treatment experience. Donahue, who acknowledged the powerful therapeutic effects of her ECT, felt unprepared for the extent of the memory loss she also experienced, as described in one of the epigraphs to this chapter:

> There is an aura of dishonesty about the side effects: discrepancies between official positions and numerous personal testimonies of more severe problems that are discounted or left unexplained. . . . My long-term memory deficits far exceed anything my doctors anticipated, I was advised about, or that are validated by research. . . . Perhaps more than anything, how could I be experiencing what I was, if all these experts were saying it wasn't so? I felt that I was being mocked by science.[7]

In a telling index of how polarizing the subject of ECT is, Donahue's account has been derided by ECT critics for its positive description of symptom relief and discounted by ECT proponents for its subjectivity.[8] In the leading contemporary textbook on ECT, Richard Abrams commented on Donahue's article, writing that "the validity of the assertions it contains is both unknown and unknowable. The sincerity of the author is not in question; the difficulty lies elsewhere, in the disjunction between objective science and subjective experience."[9] This disjunction is difficult indeed, perhaps more than Abrams allows.

What Is a "Side" Effect?

Before turning to the respective histories of these differing accounts, we should think about the meaning of the term "side effect." While the term is a deeply ingrained part of the vocabulary of biomedicine, it is comparatively new. The term's spatial language is metaphoric. By "side," we mean "not main or central," in the same way that a "side" of fries is ancillary to the main meal. We don't order fries and have a "cheeseburger on the side." But unlike side dishes of meals, side effects of therapies are rarely sought. Side effects are usually unwanted effects. When therapies do have unintended benefits, those effects often occasion a new indication for the treatment. An already classic example of this is Viagra, which was originally developed to treat angina and hypertension.[10] Medical treatments for male pattern baldness also developed from unexpected side effects from hypertension medication.[11] In these cases, the effect is no longer "side," but central.

What people consider a side effect can also be culturally variable.[12] Western patients with bipolar disorder often complain about "loss of assertiveness" as a side effect of lithium therapy, but an ethnographic study of lithium in Hong Kong found that this was one of the prized therapeutic actions in a culture that values emotional restraint. Patients and healers in a given culture may not agree on what is a side effect.[13] In biomedicine side effects are usually considered to be temporally associated with the treatment, and long-term effects can be overlooked.[14] This may help account for psychiatry's ongoing problem with side effects, as many of the side effects of important psychiatric treatments—such as tardive dyskinesia from the first antipsychotics, and memory loss from ECT—are long-term problems. When Peter Kramer published his ambivalent meditation *Listening to Prozac* in 1993, he was troubled about what the drug's efficacy said about the nature of the self, and what the moral implications of "cosmetic psychopharmacology" were. He was freed to consider these questions by his perception that, compared with earlier antidepressants, Prozac had a mild side effect profile. Prozac, though, had only been on the market for six years at that time, and while it may have been safer than some predecessors, greater problems with side effects have since emerged. Healy has pointed out that the case for Prozac's mild side effect profile was promoted by companies producing SSRIs like Prozac, and that the claim had been more hype than science.[15] This resembles the history of ECT, which was developed in order to find a safer alternative to chemical convulsive therapy, and which may soon be supplanted by new therapies such as transcranial magnetic stimulation, which researchers hope will have lowered risk for adverse cognitive effects.[16]

The earliest use of the term "side effect" cited in the Oxford English Dictionary was in 1939.[17] The term is related to the rise of biomedicine, and biomedicine's emphasis on specific efficacy for specific conditions.[18] The term marks a partial eclipse of an aspect of an earlier, "heroic" model of American medicine, where dramatic effects, even negative ones, were linked to efficacy.[19] Strychnine, for example, was included in nerve tonics in the early twentieth century, and while it had some "inconsistent stimulating effects," its inclusion was "mainly for psychological reasons, exploiting the common belief that powerful poisons are powerful cures."[20] The growing success of more specific therapy led to a decline of this belief, but the cultural residue of heroic medicine is still with us, manifest in the American penchant for aggressive medical interventions.[21]

Throughout ECT's history, there have been commentators—pro- and anti-ECT, clinicians and patients—who asserted that ECT's efficacy might be due to its drama and extremity. That is, many have thought that the treatment's efficacy was more heroic than specific. Many have similarly wondered whether the ostensible "side effect" is in fact a central effect. Is memory loss the very reason ECT works? Does ECT erase traumas or memories that cause mental illness? Anti-ECT activists have often claimed that ECT "worked" by damaging the brain, but even some pro-ECT patients have had similar perceptions. For example, Sherwin Nuland, the physician and medical historian, has written an account of his own ECT, and concluded:

> It was as though the electroshock had burned away a tightly coiled network intertwined in my brain, constricting free will. And it had also incinerated so much of my recent memory that most of the relatively new reminders to think dangerous thoughts went with it. I knew even then that my short-term memory would in time return, but I was now finally able to confront the remaining obsessional patterns and do with them what I would.[22]

Nuland also wrote:

> At the worst of times, fearful thoughts have had to be burned out of my brain with great jolts of electricity.[23]

Despite Nuland's perception, scientific opinion has mostly held that whatever ECT's mechanism of efficacy may be, it is not likely to be the memory loss, because no studies of the subject have clearly shown a correlation between memory loss and symptom relief, although it might be hard to design a study that would show such a correlation.

Memory Loss from ECT—A History of the Clinical Science

In 2007, a major figure in ECT research, Harold Sackeim, was the lead author of an article about a large and important study of cognitive effects of ECT.[24] The authors noted, "Despite ongoing controversy, there has never [before] been a large-scale, prospective study of the cognitive effects of convulsive therapy." Large-scale, prospective studies are highly valued in clinical science, and for good reason. The article presented a number of conclusions that should be of great interest to ECT practitioners and their patients. They confirmed, for example, that technique matters for reducing side effects. The electrical wave form used mattered, with sine wave stimulation causing a slowing of reaction time six months after treatment compared to brief pulse. Electrode placement mattered, bilateral ECT resulting in significantly more severe and lasting retrograde amnesia than right unilateral, and extent of retrograde amnesia due to bilateral placement directly related to the number of treatments.[25] But they also noted that many, perhaps most, sites administering ECT were using bilateral, sine wave ECT, probably because of widespread belief that this was most effective.[26] But here another finding was significant—they concluded that if dosage is carefully titrated to an individual's seizure threshold, right unilateral ECT, delivered with an ultrabrief pulse stimulation, is as effective as bilateral sine wave ECT.

As interesting as these findings are, I want to focus on where the study fits into the decades of unfolding research on ECT and cognitive effects. By several measures, the study was a methodological advance over many previous ones. I have already noted its scale, and its prospective design. Additionally, as the authors note, empirical information about ECT's long-term effects derived mainly from small sample studies conducted in research settings, with follow-up intervals frequently limited to two months or less. In other words, only recently was research on ECT beginning to attempt prospective studies with long-term follow-up—nearly 70 years since the introduction of ECT, and despite high levels of controversy about the therapy and its adverse effects. By itself, this should make any very confident claims about either the safety or the danger of ECT suspect.

Centuries before ECT proper was developed, experiments by Benjamin Franklin and contemporaries had already suggested that electric shocks to the cranium could relieve symptoms of melancholia and other mental maladies—and that the shocks could create memory disruptions.[27] Shortly after ECT was developed, research into memory loss from ECT began to appear, as early as 1941.[28] Some early studies found memory loss and others did not. Those that did claim to find memory loss cited subjective complaints strikingly similar to those cited in more recent memoirs; those that claimed none made scientific objections to claims of memory loss similar to those made today.

Almost none of the studies published in the early years of the treatment would pass muster by our highest contemporary standards of clinical evidence. Most of them had a small number of subjects, and very few were randomized or controlled. In a 1943 article, Nolan Lewis wrote one of the first articles claiming that ECT was effective because of the memory loss.[29] Lewis was director of the New York State Psychiatric Institute, and had been introduced to ECT firsthand by Kalinowsky.[30] Lewis was enthusiastic about ECT as an improvement over Metrazol because "no disagreeable sensations or effects are experienced by the patient,"[31] suggesting that he did not consider memory loss to be disagreeable. This is not as odd as it sounds. Many physicians at the time found any adverse effects from ECT mild, at least in comparison with the dread inspired by Metrazol.

Lewis disavowed interest in statistical study of the matter, on the grounds that "statistical treatment of doubtful material is seldom if ever helpful,"[32] a phrase that illustrates how dramatically standards of clinical evidence have changed. Lewis proposed that shock therapies "seem to operate therapeutically with the amnesia aiding the patients to forget their emotional problems temporarily and thus eventually breaking up the psychopathic pattern."[33] This was speculative, but there was no more convincing explanation of

ECT's efficacy. As we have seen, some early studies of ECT took a psycho-analytic view; one wondered to what extent memory losses might in fact be a species of repression, with more traumatic memories more likely to be lost.[34] Another contemporary replied that if this were the case, it would be hard to explain why more recent memories seemed more affected.[35]

M. B. Brody used case notes to support the possibility of memory loss from ECT.[36] The patients in Brody's article described losses such as the inability to recognize friends and acquaintances following ECT treatments; one of the patients was an avid traveler and had lost any trace of memory of several places she had visited. These kinds of complaints run through sub-jective accounts of ECT treatment throughout the therapy's history. While some of the patients in Brody's article were describing deficits shortly after the treatment, and reported some improvement in the months after, Brody was explicit that some of the losses remained after years and appeared to be permanent. Note also that all the patients in his report were those who had had significant recovery from their illness.

One of the most influential sources on ECT was Kalinowsky and Hoch's 1946 textbook *Shock Treatments,*[37] which denied any permanent memory loss, claiming that its possibility had been disproven. To account for the impression of memory loss, Kalinowsky and Hoch mainly referred to the "neurotic" and "hypochondriacal" characters of the patients who com-plain.[38] Although this depiction provided an alternative explanation for the impression of memory loss—an alternative, that is, to the possibility that the loss was real—Kalinowsky and Hoch did not make clear the basis for their certainty. They certainly did not present any data of a more rigorous kind than studies that did support the existence of permanent memory loss.

Several years later, in 1950, Irving Janis offered what was probably at that time the most systematic study of the question.[39] Janis noted that most studies showed that the only lasting effect of the treatment was the symp-tom relief. Janis wondered whether many reports of memory loss may have referred to losses that the patient would have experienced without the treat-ment. Despite this speculation, of the 19 patients and 11 controls in his study, the patients showed significantly more amnesia than the controls. There were two other important findings in Janis's study. The first was that, although his follow-up was only for a few months after the treatment, he did find that what memory losses there were did last. Secondly, Janis's was one of the first studies to claim that there was no correlation between memory loss and clinical improvement. This theme was developed by Borje Cronholm and Jan-Otto Ottoson, two prolific and influential ECT research-ers.[40] One of their papers was among the earliest to find that strong clini-cal improvement actually predicted less memory loss, thus questioning the hypothesis that ECT worked by causing memory loss.[41]

During the 1960s research attention turned increasingly to unilateral placement as a method to reduce the risk of memory loss.[42] A number of studies from this period had positive results and helped pave the way for unilateral placement to become a common method. In the years since, unilateral placement has often been considered to be a safer alternative, but one that might be less effective; some recent work has held that there is no loss of efficacy.[43]

By the mid-1960s, some risk of memory loss was treated as a commonplace in ECT research. One review article, for example, asserted that "ever since ECT was first used, it has been noted that an adverse effect on memory is an almost invariable sequel."[44] For example, these studies also made critical distinctions between types of memory loss.[45] The methodological weaknesses of previous studies were increasingly bemoaned, and more studies were done that attempted to meet improving standards of rigor. In 1970, for example, there was a published study comparing the effects of bilateral and unilateral ECT, which noted a number of flaws in previous studies: the strength and duration of electrical current were not held constant; randomization was not achieved; double-blindedness was not achieved; patient characteristics such as age and treatment history were not held constant; too little information was provided about the memory tests; and the measures of therapeutic improvement were not defined rigorously.[46] Although admitting to some methodological weaknesses of their own study, the authors concluded that unilateral stimulation to the non-dominant hemisphere of the brain was a "favourable modification."[47] They did not, however, look at permanent retrograde amnesia, and lamented that "it has often been pointed out that long-term response to treatment should be investigated as well as assessment of immediate response. This is partly because of the high frequency of relapse often noted after treatment . . ."[48] But with ECT use declining in the 1960s,[49] and increasing excitement about the possibilities of psychopharmacology for both psychoses and affective disorders, research into ECT's adverse effects was not at the top of the agenda for psychiatric research.

Research in the late 1970s and early 1980s continued to focus on how to minimize damage, with electrode placement a major variable considered. One 1972 article by Rhea Dornbush took it for granted that memory damage was a possible outcome of ECT, and actually speculated that unilateral electrode placement might be more harmful.[50] But Dornbush also thought the research was highly inconclusive, because of the failure to carefully distinguish among types of memory function, and to control for different ECT techniques. Another review essay a few years later maintained, on the contrary, that unilateral was indeed safer.[51] But yet again, the inconclusive state of the research was cited, the authors noting that, among other problems, there was little agreement among researchers about what measures of memory should be used, and also that most studies had compared types of ECT, rather than ECT with no ECT, so it was hard to know whether unilateral produced memory effects greater than normal forgetting.[52] But by the early 1980s, the greater safety of unilateral placement was asserted in influential publications.[53] There was also at this time some support for brief-pulse application as a safer treatment than sine wave.[54]

Larry Squire, a major memory researcher, was the lead author on a series of articles in the 1970s and 1980s that would become among the most cited publications in the study of adverse effects of ECT.[55] The work of Squire and his collaborators produced a number of results that became established premises in subsequent research. These included the findings that retrograde memory loss from ECT would be greatest for newer memories (that is, those closest in time to the treatment),[56] and that many patients could expect gradual return of memory functioning over the course of the months following the treatment.[57] This body of research did not find positively for permanent retrograde losses, but allowed for its possibility.[58]

Squire was also among a number of researchers at that time who attempted to look more rigorously at the problem of whether memory disturbances should be attributed to the presenting illness, rather than to the ECT. In one study he provided a partial setback to this view:

> Memory complaints that occurred 1 week after ECT differed quantitatively and qualitatively from memory complaints that occurred before ECT. Six months later, memory complaints qualitatively resembled the complaints reported 1 week after ECT and differed sharply from those reported before ECT. It was suggested that a patient's impression of his memory is altered by bilateral ECT and that this altered impression persists in gradually diminishing form for at least 6 months after a typical course of treatment . . . in depressed elderly patients memory complaints appeared to be related more to degree of depression than to performance on memory tests. . . . Conversely, patients receiving electroconvulsive therapy . . . who were clinically improved often denied memory impairment despite the fact that memory impairment could be documented by formal testing.[59]

Elsewhere Squire and Slater asserted that memory losses from ECT were well beyond what one would expect from depression alone.[60] And Trevor Price asserted similarly that, although depression can cause memory losses, "the memory impairments resulting from ECT tend to be just the reverse of those associated with depression."[61]

On the eve of the increase in ECT use that began in the 1980s, there was concern from within the profession that, aside from the well-established temporary memory problems, there was a possibility of permanent losses. A fascinating 1980 article on patient experiences and attitudes in the *British Journal of Psychiatry* expressed surprise at the large number of patients in the study who complained of memory losses; 30% of them complained that it never returned to normal, although 12% said it was improved.[62] One article from 1982 found that memory losses were not necessarily confined in time to the period close to the treatment,[63] and another documented long-term retrograde losses.[64] And in a study with unusually long-term follow-up, Squire and Slater found that three years after treatment, about half of the patients reported poor memory.[65] No study could claim then to be conclusive—and none did.

The need for a comprehensive review of the problem was acknowledged, and one was undertaken by Richard Weiner and published in 1984.[66] This publication had the rare accompaniment of an open peer commentary section. Weiner began by citing surveys that showed that most patients did not regard the treatment as more noxious than going to the dentist, but that brain-disabling effects had been widely publicized. He also stressed the importance of the question by re-affirming the evidence for ECT's therapeutic efficacy. Weiner claimed that most of the studies thus far had indicated that permanent memory loss was rare, but he also conceded that none of the studies were definitive. He counseled clinicians to describe permanent memory loss as possible, but rare. Most of the commentators praised Weiner for his balance, but he was condemned by prominent ECT critic Peter Breggin for going too far in denying the possibility of memory loss, and by prominent ECT proponent Max Fink for allowing its possibility. Breggin noted that there were detectable effects on the brain from ECT; Weiner countered in his response that effects on the brain do not necessarily indicate "damage" (indeed, it is hard to imagine a psychiatric treatment, including talk therapy, that could not in principle be found to have effects on the brain, as the brain is the organ that should be affected by psychiatric treatment).[67] Weiner lamented that there were reasons many people might find Breggin's argument persuasive, including sensationalist media treatments of ECT, past abuses of the treatment, and poor technique continuing to lead to cognitive deficits. Fink felt the burden of proof ought to be on those who would claim cognitive losses from ECT, a view Weiner expressed ambivalence toward. Weiner wrote that "in a way, this view has merit, since . . . the null hypothesis, that is, that no brain damage occurs with ECT, is impossible to prove with 100% certainty. An argument can always be made, for example, that the memory tests were not sufficiently sensitive, that the anatomic regions studied were not sufficiently widespread, that the wrong biochemical constituents were assayed, and so on . . ."[68] Still, Weiner also found Fink's argument overly legalistic and feared that it could have the effect of stifling further research. Squire emphasized that review articles can support almost anything, because one can almost always find the studies that support one's point of view. Squire—a notable voice for empirical caution throughout these debates—concluded that permanent memory losses from ECT were neither proven nor unproven.

As we have seen, some acknowledged risk of memory losses resulting from mental illnesses has raised doubt about whether to attribute losses to the treatment. As research progressed in the 1980s and 1990s, evidence grew that losses were due to the treatment, even if illness also contributed.

For example, a 1994 study suggested that there were identifiable differences between the losses due to depression and those due to the treatment:

> The ratings that worsened most from pre- to posttreatment were thought to result from complaints due to ECT itself, while those memory difficulties that remained unchanged might be due to some residual depression. The complaints that worsened involved remembering names, faces, and past events, e.g., 'My ability to search through my mind and recall names and memories I know are there is . . .' The complaints that were attributed to depression dealt with general alertness, ability to pay attention, understand instructions . . .[69]

A 1989 study compared bilaterally treated ECT patients with patients treated with the antidepressant imipramine.[70] The ECT patients showed better improvement from their illness, but experienced memory losses not seen in patients treated with imipramine:

> Both ECT- and imipramine-treated patients showed a deficit in recent anterograde memory relative to their pretreatment performance . . . ECT-treated patients also had a significant and well-characterized impairment in retrograde remote memory. By contrast, imipramine-treated patients did not show a retrograde memory impairment which could be explained by treatment.

More recent research has continued to consider various variables influencing the extent of memory loss from ECT. A 1985 study found that greater seizure duration was a risk factor for memory loss.[71] A 1986 study found evidence for personal memory losses lasting at least six months with bilateral treatment but not with unilateral.[72] A 1995 study cautiously suggested that while anterograde memory disturbance does gradually clear up in the months after ECT, there is the possibility of lasting retrograde losses.[73] A study in 2000 found that ECT patients lost more memories than controls, with deficits more marked for impersonal than personal items, bilateral more than right unilateral, and added that although memories "usually" return, memories do not return for "many" patients.[74] Still, despite a number of studies finding risk of long-term or permanent losses, there continued to be a number of publications that considered the data inconclusive, or supporting safety. One study found an absence of cognitive effects in patients who had had more than 100 treatments in a lifetime, but this study had a very small sample, with eight patients and eight controls.[75]

Among the most important writing by a clinical researcher was not a scientific study, but an editorial by psychologist and ECT researcher Harold Sackeim in the journal *Convulsive Therapy* in 2000.[76] Although not a research article, it carried authority because Sackeim is among the most prominent ECT experts, known to be highly conversant with the state of the literature. Noting the polarization between critics who maintain that efficacy is an illusion fostered by the "punch-drunk" quality of the patients, and supporters who deny any lasting cognitive deficits from ECT, Sackeim countered both. On the one hand, he noted that studies had shown no correlation between deficits and symptom relief. On the other hand, Sackeim wrote that *"virtually all* patients experience some degree of persistent and likely permanent retrograde amnesia."[77] This was a startling claim, given that many clinicians and clinical textbooks describe ECT as very safe. While acknowledging that complaints about memory loss may be subjective, Sackeim countered claims that complaints of memory loss were hysterical by noting that "there is no dearth of patients who have received ECT who believe that the treatment was valuable, often life saving, who are not litigious, who return to productive activities, and yet report that a large segment of their life is lost."[78] In fact, as we will see later in this article, the narrative evidence is replete with stories that fit this description.

As Hirshbein has emphasized, a history of the science certainly shows that there has also been no dearth of study on ECT and memory loss.[79] Decades of study have shown that there is some risk. The question has been studied from many angles, such as variations in technique, and attempts to control for the effects of the illness. But on a key question—how common are retrograde losses?—I do not believe we have a scientific consensus or even a great deal of data. As a contrast, one could point to the scientific literature on the efficacy of ECT for providing symptom relief, on which the scientific consensus is robust. Many of the greatest detractors of ECT practice concede its efficacy.

Recall here both the certainty with which many clinicians assert that all the lost memories return, and some of the statements in widely known handbooks and textbooks of ECT. Max Fink, one of the physicians most responsible for promoting the revival of ECT, has written an account for lay readers that asserts that "the procedure [is] so safe that the risks are less than those which accompany the use of several psychotropic drugs,"[80] and that

> the prevalent belief that electroshock impairs memory is based on the early experiences of patients who were treated without anesthesia or ventilation with oxygen. Such treatments were associated with severe and persistent memory losses. There is no longer any validity to the fear that electroshock will erase memory or make the patient unable to recall her life's important events or recognize family members or return to work.[81]

As I mentioned elsewhere in the book, Fink quotes a patient who thought ECT was no worse than a trip to the dentist. One does not, though, expect to forget major life events or close acquaintances after a teeth cleaning. Richard Abrams, author of a leading clinical textbook on ECT, as well as a manufacturer of ECT devices, did a thorough review of studies of ECT and cognition.[82] Abrams recognized the existence of subjective complaints of memory loss as a result of the treatment, and acknowledged that the subjective complaints *might* be valid, but asserted that there was no convincing objective data to prove it. But the reverse is also true: the case for the rarity of permanent memory loss is unproven. A prominent handbook for clinicians similarly asserts that permanent memory loss, while unfortunate, is very rare.[83] One of the co-authors of this handbook has elsewhere argued that being honest about ECT means acknowledging that in addition to its powerful therapeutic effects, it has serious side effects.[84]

Narrative Accounts

This section looks closely at representations of memory loss in narrative accounts of ECT. Memory loss does not feature universally in these accounts. From Frank Kimball (Chapter Two) to Norman Endler (Chapter Five), there have been patients who have touted healing effect without any lament over lost memory. Nevertheless, given how rare permanent losses are held to be in much of the scientific literature, it is striking how common they are in narrative accounts. To avoid a possible misunderstanding: I will not be claiming that narrative evidence proves that claims for the rarity of memory loss are wrong. I am, though, claiming that laments about memory loss in narrative accounts are so frequent, and appear in accounts that differ so widely by other measures that, minimally, they pose a puzzle: the question of whether scientific study has been adequately capturing them.

Surprisingly, memory loss features most prominently in more recent accounts. This is ironic, because technical innovations in ECT treatment have been intended to reduce cognitive side effects, and research in the scientific studies indicates that they have. One reason why these claims are rarer in the earlier accounts may be that early ECT often had features that were more upsetting than memory loss. Complaints about ECT in the first decades of its use focused on the fear of the treatment, and its involuntary use. Another reason there are not many narrative accounts of memory loss is that narrative accounts of any kind were more rare. In the 1940s and 1950s, it was simply less common for people to write and publish stories of their illnesses than it would later become. We know, nevertheless, that some patients were reporting memory losses in the early years of ECT, because clinicians were taking the trouble to study the problem.

One famous and early account was by Ernest Hemingway, who was, shortly before his suicide, treated with ECT for long-standing struggles with madness.[85] Hemingway was very bitter about the amnesias he experienced, and famously said, "Well, what is the sense of ruining my head and erasing my memory, which is my capital, and putting me out of business? It was a brilliant cure but we lost the patient." One might wonder whether Hemingway's suicide was due to his distress at the side effects of the treatment, although here we face a conundrum common to any case of a suicide follow-ing a treatment for mental illness, as the suicide could as logically be attrib-uted to the mental illness. According to Hemingway biographer Kenneth Lynn, Hemingway actually did experience some short-lived symptom relief from the ECT, including improved mood and restored sex drive, although Mary Welsh, Hemingway's third wife, thought his Mayo Clinic doctors botched the case, because they considered him more improved than he was. Regardless of how improved he was, he blamed the ECT for compromising his writing ability, although those abilities had likely been, by Hemingway's own estimation, in decline for years before the ECT.

Rock star Lou Reed was treated with ECT when he was young, before he was famous. Some accounts claim that his parents made him undergo psychiatric treatment out of fear that he was gay, but his sister has said that he was suffering from severe anxiety and depression at the time, and that his parents were not at all homophobic.[86] Reed received ECT, and then complained of memory problems that seem to have been more anterograde than retrograde:

> They put the thing down your throat so you don't swallow your tongue, and they put electrodes on your head. That's what was recommended in Rockland County to discourage homosexual feelings. The effect is that you lose your memory and become a vegetable. You can't read a book because you get to page seventeen and have to go right back to page one again.[87]

Reed's reference to becoming a "vegetable" is of course a standard, cultur-ally available image for adverse effects of ECT treatment. There is some irony in it being voiced by a man who went on to become one of the most creative forces in the history of rock music—one whose great 1982 album "The Blue Mask" can be read as a powerful depiction of the pain of depres-sion. Velvet Underground bandmate John Cale said that every time Reed told the story of his time in a mental hospital, the details changed.[88] Cale's testimony explicitly casts doubt on Reed's, but it may implicitly support Reed's view that his memory was damaged.

Judith Kruger's 1959 memoir of her recovery from mental illness also lamented memory loss.[89] Unlike many similar memoirs, Kruger's account contains little description of the onset of the illness. Like many ECT patients, Kruger felt mounting fear as the treatment drew nearer, and she had actually heard that ECT could cause memory loss. Kruger depicts a clear sense of relief at the remission of her symptoms after some treatment. She describes a general sense of calm, and an ability to sleep restfully for the first time in weeks. This relief did not translate into any enthusiasm for the procedure, though. In fact, the word she used to describe her feelings toward it was "hate."[90] And this is understandable, because although her account does not provide enough technical detail to know what kind of

ECT she received or whether she had general anesthesia, she did experience the outward convulsions that were characteristic of early ECT practice.[91] Her ire was also directed at memory loss, though: "I stood in the shower naked in body and mind. I couldn't recall the date, or the baby's name, or who was with him at home."[92] She felt that the memory loss worsened with successive treatments, adding: "It's like waking up from the nowhere into anywhere."[93]

Kruger's evocative writing about the impairments provides insight into why many patients who are helped by ECT also dislike it. But her book is limited to the time of her treatment, so the memory loss depicted does not address any controversy over long-term or permanent impairments. There are memoirs, though, that are more suggestive of permanent losses.

One such is Ellen Wolfe's *Aftershock*.[94] Wolfe (a pseudonym) had been in psychotherapy for what she herself regarded as a low-level common case of neurosis, and then one day woke up in the hospital, where she was told she had had a "nervous breakdown." Descriptions of her illness suggest a severe manic episode with psychotic features, although her account contains little description of the "descent." In fact, she forgot much of it.

Wolfe's memory losses included forgetting the existence of her second child, a daughter, as well as public events such as the assassination of President Kennedy, whom she thought was still president. Her husband also needed to remind her that she had had an abortion prior to the episode that resulted in her hospitalization. At a number of points, Wolfe referred to the humiliation felt upon not remembering an acquaintance after her ECT, a theme echoed in many patient accounts of ECT. She described her memory loss as being like "waking up—*but all day long.*"[95]

Clinicians frequently assured Wolfe and her husband that all her memories would return, but her narrative—which appears to have been written some time after the treatment—ends with her still lamenting the memory loss. Her doctors also encouraged her to stop worrying about the memory loss and move on, but Wolfe's response shows why memory loss is so troubling: "Forget about the past? We *are* the past."[96] Put another way, memory loss is a frightening effect because memory is held to be identical with the self.[97] Wolfe at no point questions the therapeutic efficacy of the ECT. Any gratitude for it may have been blunted, though, by her lack of memory for the illness itself. Wolfe actually regretted the very speed with which the ECT returned her to normalcy, as it deprived her of time in the sick role.[98]

Wolfe's account is cited in several clinical studies. One prominent ECT practitioner, Charles Kellner, has stressed his own impression that Wolfe's memory complaints do not appear to his experienced clinical eye to have been "hysterical" in origin.[99] That is, Kellner saw no sign that the complaints were without organic basis, although he did speculate that they may have been due at least partly to the severity of her illness, and partly to the use of bilateral application of the ECT.

Marion Milner's *The Hands of the Living God* appeared the same year as *Aftershock*.[100] Written by the patient's psychoanalyst, *The Hands of the Living God* dwells at length on the patient's subjective reaction to ECT—which in this case is especially complicated by the patient's severe psychopathology, with elements of psychosis both before and after the ECT. *The Hands of the Living God* does not mention memory loss, as such. It does, however, describe at length the patient's sensation that the ECT took away her self or her soul. As Milner put it, she felt that "since the E.C.T., she had no inner world nor internal perceptions."[101]

This theme of inner emptiness was echoed several years later in an account by Burton Roueché in the *New Yorker*.[102] Roueché's subject was identified by the pseudonym "Natalie Parker" in the article, and is now known to have been Marilyn Rice, who became an important activist and critic of ECT. Rice reportedly began experiencing depression when some poorly done dental procedures transformed her into what she considered to be an ugly woman. A stay in a mental hospital, which she did not remember, caused severe damage to her memory. As she put it: "Now I know how Eve must have felt, having been created full grown out of somebody's rib without any past history. I feel as empty as Eve."[103] Rice also said: "Somebody the other day asked me to make a fourth at bridge and I refused saying I hadn't played bridge for at least fifteen years. Then he said I had been playing right along for the two months I had been at the hospital."[104] Roueché noted that "Mrs. Parker's return . . . to the apartment that had been her home for many years was something of a *déjà-vu* experience. She had an uncertain feeling that she had been there before."[105] And finally, as Rice emphasized, "There weren't just gaps in my memory. There were oceans and oceans of blankness."[106] Aspects of her story, like forgetting the bridge games, would count among the memory problems associated with the time of the treatment, and thus would be considered normal by most ECT clinicians. Rice, though, considered herself to have very significant long-term losses, and this is why she became an anti-ECT activist.

Similar "blankness" was a major theme in Robert Pirsig's popular 1974 meditation *Zen and the Art of Motorcycle Maintenance*. Pirsig's book is an unusual one in its combination of memoir and philosophical reflection. Pirsig states at the outset that much of the book is fictionalized—"changed for rhetorical purposes"—but readers are urged to consider it "in its essence as fact."[107] It is hard to know whether any particular assertions or descriptions in the book should be taken as factual or rhetorical. We know from other sources that Pirsig did suffer from a breakdown of some kind, and received ECT. In the book, the treatment figures as a dividing line between the life of "Phaedrus," a previous version of his self, but one with which he has such a poor connection in memory that another name is needed for him. The descriptions are, at times, reminiscent of Wolfe's in that places and situations feel oddly familiar, but the reason for their familiarity feels elusive:

There, out the window in the dark—this cold wind crossing the road into the trees, the leaves shimmering flecks of moonlight—there is no question about it, Phaedrus saw all of this. What he was doing here I have no idea. Why he came this way I will probably never know. But he has been here, steered us onto this strange road, has been with us all along. There is no escape.[108]

Pirsig's treatment, described in the book as "annihilation EST," appears to have been the especially intense form of convulsive therapy associated with Ewen Cameron. This form of ECT was unusual, so even if understood as a factual account of Pirsig's life, his memory losses need to be understood in this context.

The stories related by Wolfe, Roueché, and Pirsig were in many ways of a piece with the antipsychiatry popular then, and which was dramatized in fictional accounts like *One Flew Over the Cuckoo's Nest*. Starting in the 1980s, a very different tone began to be struck in published memoirs of ECT. These were not the first published accounts of ECT that were positive, but a growing number of patients were beginning to provide accounts that stressed beneficial effects. For example, Endler's *Holiday of Darkness,* which appeared in 1982, chronicled the author's gradual acceptance that he was suffering from depression, and subsequent gratitude for the symptom relief provided by ECT—a treatment he had been professionally hostile to prior to his own depression. But many of these new narratives did not deny serious side effects. Actually, the descriptions of memory loss in these narratives are quite as vivid as those in the very negative portrayals. The difference is rather that in the newer stories, the lament over memory loss is often mingled with equally vivid gratitude for symptom relief. This makes their testimony about memory loss highly credible; one cannot easily dismiss these accounts as the work of antipsychiatric cranks.

Andrew Solomon's wide-ranging exploration of depression, *The Noon-Day Demon,* contains few accounts of ECT treatments, but permanent memory loss is related in every single one of them.[109] Solomon tells the story, for example, of Bill Stein, who had had a number of serious depressions before a severe episode in 1986 led him to seek ECT.[110] Stein's problems appear to be at least partly anterograde; he told Solomon,

> I still mourn the loss of my memory . . . I had an exceptional memory, nearly photographic, and it has never come back. When I got out [of the hospital] I couldn't remember my locker combination, my conversations. . . . Perhaps it is just as well that my memory was clearly suffering permanent deficits. . . . It has helped me to blunt out some of the lows.[111]

Stein felt Prozac to be a salvation, which "came along in 1988, just in time" to help him manage his mood. Solomon also relates the case of a prominent lawyer who emerged from her ECT treatment with no recollection of law school; Solomon calls cases like this rare and extreme—presumably on the basis of his reading of the clinical literature—although there is not in his book a case of ECT that does not involve significant memory loss.[112] The third case he describes is Frank Rusakoff, who expresses displeasure from memory problems even as he calls the treatment safe:

> ECT works, but I hate it. It's totally safe and I would recommend it, but they're putting electricity into your head, and that's scary. I hate the memory problems. It gives me a headache. I'm always afraid they'll do something wrong, or I won't come out of it. I keep journals so I can remember what happened; otherwise I'd never know.[113]

Martha Manning's *Undercurrents* is a defense of ECT, and her own decision to have it.[114] Certainly anti-ECT activists have taken it that way, and condemned Manning for it.[115] Manning credited ECT with relieving a depression that was resistant to psychotherapy and medication. She describes deep apprehension prior to the treatment, a consciousness that a treatment to the brain was on the face of it a threat to cognition and memory and therefore to the self.[116] Manning's account does not dwell at length in memory loss, but she does notice it in, for example, completely having forgotten a novel—Jeanette Winterson's *The Passion*—that she read before the treatment—forgetting, that is, not just the plot or the characters (as I did), but the very fact of having read it.[117] She also describes some anterograde memory problems, such as forgetting the visit of her sister one day after the visit.[118] She did not, therefore, deny adverse effects. The overwhelming impression from the book is that she simply found them an acceptable price of recovery.

Donahue's account appeared in 2000. Donahue described losing memories of having met prominent people such as Mother Theresa and Colin Powell. These are episodic memories of events likely to be emotionally powerful, and unlikely to have been lost as a matter of the normal course of life. Probably more devastating were her losses of memories of more personal things. Memory losses, she wrote,

> affected my relationships with newer, more casual friends in a different way. I simply did not remember the status of our relationship. . . . I was not prepared to discuss ECT with them, and without being able to explain uncertain overtures, I was not comfortable approaching them. Most of these friends knew basically about my illness, and would have waited to hear from me, not wanting to intrude. The relationships with these people basically drifted away.[119]

Donahue also described not knowing why she had had stitches in her forehead (it was from a fall in 1994), and needing to learn not to rely on her memory: "I have to keep vigilant to not prejudge someone as lying or misleading simply because I forgot that the fault could have been my memory. . . . Sometimes it gave me a sense of being an outsider looking in to my own past world."[120]

Donahue—who not only acknowledged the therapeutic benefits of the ECT, but said she would still have had it if she had known she would have the memory loss—was especially bitter about what she felt was inadequate preparation for the side effects:

> I had in fact experienced significant and long-term impairment that I could *easily* distinguish from ordinary memory fallibility. Yet as I reviewed what I had found, it seemed clear that comprehensive efforts to assess long-term severe adverse effects had not been made. *I found repeated acknowledgment that more research was needed on memory loss* . . .[121]

It is important to underscore that Donahue does not regard herself as opposed to ECT. In another article, she describes having been prescribed a number of other treatments for major depression, but says that it was only with the ECT that her recovery began.[122]

Andy Behrman's account of his ECT is very enthusiastic about therapeutic benefits, yet strikingly similar to Donahue's in his description of memory difficulties.[123] Behrman wrote:

> After four treatments, there is marked improvement [in his symptoms of bi-polar disorder]. No more egregious highs or lows. But there are huge gaps in my memory. I avoid friends and neighbors because I don't know their names anymore. I can't remember the books I've read or the movies I've seen. I have trouble recalling simple vocabulary. I forget phone numbers. Sometimes I even forget what floor I live on. It's embarrassing. But I continue treatment because I'm getting better.[124]

Another account by a recent patient with bipolar disorder is Terri Cheney's *Manic*.[125] A gripping and best-selling account of illness, Cheney's book, like many recent accounts, mingles recognition of symptom relief with lamentation over memory loss. Some passages read as though they could be featured in promotion brochures for ECT:

> Before the ECT, the world had been a dull and muddy gray, with strains of funeral black. Now it was raucous and bright as a tropical parrot, and just as exotic. I seemed to hear things I'd never heard before: one leaf rustling up against another, the insinuating whisper of the wind.[126]
>
> I thought back to the face I'd seen in my bathroom mirror before the ECT: sullen, sallow, the smile muscles slack from disuse. And I looked at me now: pink-cheeked and blooming, trembling with anticipation, every pore, every freckle alive and alert.[127]

But despite the evident torture her illness has been, Cheney definitely considered ECT to have serious costs:

> The ECT may have kicked me out of the depression, but it kicked a little too hard. Not only did I lose most of my inhibitions, I lost a good part of my memory, too. I could remember some things well enough . . . but I completely forgot basic essential info like what different utensils were for. I happily ate my ice cream with a fork, my fish with a spoon. I forgot standard social etiquette, too, like the custom of shaking hands upon meeting someone.[128]
>
> ECT can be of great help as a last-resort treatment, but it's notorious for wiping out memory. For a while, I forgot even the simplest things: what part of town I lived in, my mother's maiden name, what scissors were for. Some of this was eventually restored, but I still have trouble recalling past events and retaining memories of new ones. The world has never seemed as sharp and clear as it did before ECT.[129]

Cheney acknowledges some restoration of the lost memory, but judges that much or most of it was permanent.

Writer Jonathan Cott's experience with ECT led him to produce an extended meditation on the nature of memory.[130] He received 36 ECT treatments for depression, and although he acknowledged the possible role of confounds such as stress, aging, and the depression itself, he said with decisive certainty that ECT permanently erased innumerable memories.[131] His described losses included both personal and impersonal, retrograde and anterograde, and included the end of the Cold War, the end of apartheid, famous people who died during the period of the losses (which included Princess Diana, Glenn Gould, and John Lennon), favorite books read during this period, and even the research and writing of six books and a number of magazine articles, which seemed "as though written by someone else."[132] He also describes aphasia, problems remembering items he had just read, and a gradual loss of the knowledge of the content of films recently seen, with the endings going first, then the middle, and finally the beginnings.[133] Cott's account is among the more critical of recent accounts. He researched the history and science of ECT, and concluded that there were too many statements by prominent psychiatrists that downplayed the risk of adverse effects, and lax regulation by the federal government of ECT. Still, Cott is not among the abolitionists, and he also criticized ECT detractors who went on to indiscriminate condemnation of psychiatry. Despite his mourning over his own losses, he acknowledged ECT's power to relieve symptoms, and supported its use as a last-resort treatment.

Another recent account is in Carrie Fisher's wry memoir *Shockaholic*.[134] Like many ECT memoirs, Fisher's includes a recollection of imagining the worst about ECT because of cinematic portrayals. Fisher found her ECT therapeutic, and as her title suggests, she has gone back for voluntary repeat treatments, describing the power of ECT to effect change on her previously intractable affective disorder: "And whereas before my brain had felt as though it was set in cement, leaving me . . . I don't know . . . kind of stuck, the ECT blasted my Hoover Dam head wide open, moving the immoveable."[135] But Fisher described both retrograde and anterograde losses, and concluded that "the truly negative thing about ECT is that it's incredibly hungry and the only thing it has a taste for is memory."[136] It is striking, given the complaints about memory loss, that Fisher has returned for voluntary repeat treatments.

There is no question that more unequivocally negative accounts of ECT treatment continue to appear. Linda Andre's *Doctors of Deception* is both one such account, as well as itself a history of ECT.[137] Andre gives powerful voice to those who have felt the procedure was either forced on them, or who felt pressured into the treatment without adequate information about adverse effects.

Patients who do not report symptom relief or who might not have even thought of themselves as needing a powerful treatment to begin with are rightly troubled about ECT. But the accounts that commingle descriptions of relief from symptoms and grieving for lost memory constitute a powerful form of evidence, precisely because one would not expect a patient subjectively helped by her treatment to emphasize adverse effects if they did not have compelling reason to think they occurred.

The foregoing accounts of memory loss are disquieting regardless of how representative they are. Memory is so dear, one will want to know of the chance of losing it, even if the chance is small. One might ask of these published stories questions of selection bias, though. Are unhappy patients more likely to write or get published? Are patients with memory loss more motivated to write and publish their story? Or are publishers more interested in these accounts? Is there, in other words, a vast silent majority of satisfied ECT patients who have suffered little or no permanent memory loss? There are several reasons why it would be hazardous to assume that a selection bias accounts for the frequency of descriptions of memory loss. Accounts that depict memory loss are, as I have stressed, by no means all characterized by bitterness and opposition to the treatment. Memory loss is as likely to be to be portrayed in narratives that openly endorse ECT as a treatment as in those that oppose it. It is even possible that patients with the most memory loss are among the least likely to produce accounts of their treatment, because they simply lack the cognitive skills.

The narrative evidence also raises doubts about some of the alternative explanations that have been offered for perceived memory losses after ECT. The depression memoir is a flourishing literary genre, and while memory loss is a ubiquitous feature of memoirs with ECT, it is relatively absent from those that lack an account of ECT treatment. For those who claim that the reported memory losses are due to the illness itself, this is an enigmatic detail to explain. While some researchers since Kalinowsky have been referring to complaints of memory loss as "hysterical," no one seems to be writing memoirs about how Prozac or Effexor destroyed their memory.[138] People on Prozac complain about headaches or impotence.

The descriptions of memory loss in these accounts cannot settle any questions about the commonness of the problems described. Not only is it hard to establish their representativeness, but many variables are often unclear in the accounts, such as what technique of ECT was used and how close the memories were to the time of the treatment. But they are important for several reasons. At a minimum, they convey the subjective experiences of believing one's memory to be badly impaired by ECT. It has also been shown that the memories lost due to ECT are qualitatively different from those lost to mental illnesses.[139] The losses are unlikely to be from other causes, with the ECT as a convenient scapegoat. Few of the memoirs, for example, are by elderly people, so senility is not a likely explanation.

No accumulation of narrative accounts will satisfy any demands for controlled, statistically significant studies. But even very rigorous scientific studies will continue to raise questions about whether they are adequately measuring the losses. Both sides of this debate have been enabled by weaknesses of their opponents' arguments. This is a problem resistant to definitive resolution. Each side has had many alternative explanations for the evidence introduced by the other. I wonder, in fact, whether any research would actually satisfy both sides of the debate,[140] although it is certainly worth trying. New technologies, such as transcranial magnetic stimulation (TMS), may render the question moot by providing comparable relief without cognitive deficits—although, if ECT is as safe as its strongest proponents suggest, it is hard to see why we should be researching or adopting TMS.

Conclusion

Decades of historiography about psychological treatments, such as psychoanalysis, have shown beyond doubt that patient experience depends on context. This makes intuitive sense; it is easy to see how a talk therapy would be grounded in culture. The historical quality of response to physical treatments may be less apparent.

We know of course that the technology can change, and this makes a difference. We also know that science changes—for example, due to intellectual fashions such as the rise and fall of psychoanalysis. But can wider cultural change have an independent effect on the experience of physical treatments? Despite a couple of decades of attempts to historicize the body, the intuition remains strong that the body is a relatively timeless given of nature.

The growing number of complaints about memory loss may be partly due to an increase in the premium placed on cognition. Several authors have shown that late twentieth-century American culture came to place a special value on cognitive ability.[141] Solomon seems to suggest that this cultural valuation accounts for the current popularity of antidepressants:

To understand the history of depression is to understand the invention of the human being as we know him and are him. Our Prozac-popping, cognitively focused, semi-alienated postmodernity is only a stage in the ongoing understanding and control of mood and character.[142]

Solomon is arguing that depression is a human constant, but one that has gone through many vagaries regarding cultural attitudes, vagaries that help to account for changing fashions in treatment. The heavy premium placed on high cognitive functioning in an advanced industrial society would help account for the high reliance on antidepressants; affective disorders may be troublesome to anyone, but are arguably less tolerable for knowledge workers whose mental faculties must be at their best for their work to be most effective. It would also help to explain the rise of two other treatments for affective disorder—cognitive therapy and ECT. All three of these (psychopharmaceuticals, cognitive therapy, and ECT) are marked by the promise of speedy release from the shackles of depression. The psychoanalysis favored in the middle of the twentieth century was, by contrast, marked by its slowness and its attention to complex emotional conflicts and the irrational. If ECT is currently valued for its speed, and its power to return the patient to functioning, it is also devalued for its cognitive side effects to a greater extent than it was in its early years. There is some reason to think that, more generally, our society has a growing intolerance for medical symptoms—we expect more from our bodies than previous generations did, in numerous areas, including longevity, physical comfort, sexual performance, and affective stability—and we expect medicine to provide solutions when our bodies do not deliver.[143] In this context, cognitive complaints such as memory loss become more troublesome effects.

Peter Breggin, in his book lambasting ECT, argued that the reason women get more ECT than men is that our society values the cognitive abilities of women less than those of men.[144] He made no attempt to control for diagnosis rates—that is, if women are diagnosed with severe depression more than men, one would expect them to get more ECT, regardless of how much one values their cognition. He also assumed psychiatrists administering ECT share his view that ECT is brain-disabling, and many do not. Still, there may be a point of interest to be taken from his perspective. It is possible that the complaints about memory loss reflect gains from feminism, as women and their loved ones are no longer willing to tolerate cognitive disturbances that once would have been accepted. It is certainly well established by historians that psychiatry, and indeed all of medicine, has a poor track record when it comes to listening to complaints about treatment from women.[145]

What emerges more definitely from the history of this side effect is one explanation for the protracted nature of the ECT debate. ECT's therapeutic power has been hard to deny. Yet on a very central question of its power to harm—the frequency of permanent memory loss—there is a substantial uncertainty.

Opponents of ECT often portray it as a barbaric throwback, comparing it to obsolete practices such as leeching or bloodletting. These comparisons are sensationalist, in that they are meant only to ridicule by creating gruesome associations, rather than making a sober assessment of the benefits and costs of the treatment. Yet these comparisons also make some symbolic sense. ECT is an unspecific treatment, and the reason for its efficacy is mysterious. In this sense, it is a heroic therapy in a post-heroic medical culture, a remnant indeed, but one whose efficacy has enabled it to survive. This further helps to explain why it has been controversial.

Notes

1 Anne B. Donahue, "Electroconvulsive Therapy and Memory Loss: A Personal Journey," *The Journal of ECT* 16, 2 (2000) 133–143. The quotes reproduced here are on pages 134 and 138.

2 Ellen Wolfe, *Aftershock: The Story of a Psychotic Episode* (New York: G.P. Putnam's and Sons, 1969), 83.

3 Joan Prudic, Shoshana Peyser, and Harold A. Sackeim, "Subjective Memory Complaints: A Review of Patient Self-Assessment of Memory after Electroconvulsive Therapy," *The Journal of ECT* 16, 2 (2000) 121–132.

4 See Richard Abrams, *Electroconvulsive Therapy* (4th edition, Oxford: Oxford University Press, 2002) ch. 10, and Charles H. Kellner, John T. Pritchett, Mark D. Beale, and C. Edward Coffey, *Handbook of ECT* (Washington, D.C.: American Psychiatric Press, 1997), 87–89.

5 On this topic, see also Laura Hirshbein, "Electroconvulsive Therapy, Memory, and Self in America," *Journal of the History of the Neurosciences: Basic and Clinical Perspectives* 21, 2 (2012) 147–169. Hirshbein refers to some of the same scientific literature as I do, but does not look at patients' accounts. Our analyses are substantially different, but more compatible than conflicting.

6 UK ECT Review Group, "Efficacy and Safety of Electroconvulsive Therapy in Depressive Disorders: A Systematic Review and Meta-Analysis," *The Lancet* 361 (March 8, 2003) 799–808.

7 Anne B. Donahue, "Electroconvulsive Therapy and Memory Loss: A Personal Journey." The quotes reproduced here are on pages 134 and 138.

8 Kitty Dukakis and Larry Tye, *Shock: The Healing Power of Electroconvulsive Therapy* (New York: Penguin, 2006), 166.

9 Abrams, *Electroconvulsive Therapy*, 200.

10 See Jennifer Fishman, "Making Viagra: From Impotence to Erectile Dysfunction," in Andrea Tone and Elizabeth Siegel Watkins, eds., *Medicating Modern America* (New York: New York University Press, 2007). Fishman stresses that this story of fortuitous discovery runs the risk of obscuring the longer history of medical research on treatments for impotence.

11 Peter Conrad, *The Medicalization of Society*, 37.

12 Nina L. Etkin, "'Side Effects': Cultural Constructions and Reinterpretations of Western Pharmaceuticals," *Medical Anthropology Quarterly* 6, 2 (1992), 99–113.

13 Etkin, "Side Effects," 102.

14 Etkin, "Side Effects," 101.

15 David Healy, *Let Them Eat Prozac: The Unhealthy Relationship between the Pharmaceutical Industry and Depression* (New York: New York University Press, 2004).

16 Sarah H. Lisanby, ed., *Brain Stimulation in Psychiatric Treatment* (Washington, D.C.: American Psychiatric Publishing, Inc., 2004).

17 *Oxford English Dictionary On-Line,* accessed July 24, 2007.

18 Etkin, "Side Effects." The attention to the problem of side effects in the 1930s may also have been related particularly to the introduction of the sulfonamides, the first effective antibacterial agents, and the toxic effects they had. See Barron Lerner, "Scientific Evidence versus Therapeutic Demand: The Introduction of the Sulfonamides Revisited," *Annals of Internal Medicine* 115 (1991) 315–320.

19 Rosenberg, "The Therapeutic Revolution."

20 Rasmussen, *On Speed,* 9.

21 Payer, *Medicine and Culture.*

22 Sherwin Nuland, *Lost in America: A Journey with My Father* (New York: Alfred A. Knopf, 2003), 7–8.

23 Nuland, *Lost in America,* 211.

24 Harold A. Sackeim, Joan Prudic, Rice Fuller, John Keilp, Philip W. Lavori, and Mark Olfson, "The Cognitive Effects of Electroconvulsive Therapy in Community Settings," *Neuropsychopharmacology* 32 (2007) 244–254.

25 Sackeim et al. "Cognitive Effects," 244. The authors were careful to stress that although technique appears to influence extent of adverse effects, their data were not robust enough to rule out adverse effects from the safer methods.

26 Sackeim et al. "Cognitive Effects," 245.

27 Stanley Finger and Franklin Zaromb, "Benjamin Franklin and Shock-Induced Amnesia," *American Psychologist* 61, 3 (April 2006) 240–248; Sherry Ann Beaudreau and Stanley Finger, "Medical Electricity and Madness in the 18th Century," *Perspectives in Biology and Medicine* 49, 3 (Summer 2006) 330–345. These eighteenth-century therapeutic experiments with shocks were most likely subconvulsive; see Beaudreau and Finger, "Medical Electricity," 343. There is also no evidence that Cerletti and Bini were influenced by these earlier electrical therapies; see Finger and Zaromb, "Benjamin Franklin," 247.

28 For example, Sherman and Mergener studied anterograde memory following ECT. The patients in the study showed no deficits, but the study had only 10 subjects. Irene Sherman and John Mergener, "The Effect of Convulsive Treatment on Memory," *American Journal of Psychiatry* 98 (November 1941) 402–403.

29 Nolan D. C. Lewis, "The Present Status of Shock Therapy of Mental Disorders," *Bulletin of the New York Academy of Medicine* (April 1943) 227–243.

30 Shorter and Healy, *Shock Therapy,* 76–77.

31 Quoted in Shorter and Healy, 77.

32 Lewis, "Present Status," 227.

33 Lewis, "Present Status," 236.

34 C. G. Holland, "The Complaint of 'Forgetting' following Electroshock," *Virginia Medical Monthly* (May 1950) 221–226.

35 Donald R. Stieper, Meyer Williams, and Carl P. Duncan, "Changes in Impersonal and Personal Memory following Electro-Convulsive Therapy," *Journal of Clinical Psychology* VII, 4 (October 1951) 361–366.

36 M. B. Brody, "Prolonged Memory Defects following Electro-Therapy," *Journal of Mental Science* 90, 380 (July 1944) 777–779.

37 Lothar B. Kalinowsky and Paul H. Hoch, *Shock Treatments.*

38 Kalinowsky and Hoch, *Shock Treatments,* 134–135. Kalinowsky would repeat these arguments in Lothar Kalinowsky, "Present Status of Electroconvulsive Therapy," *Current Psychiatric Therapies* 1 (1961) 117–124.

39 Irving L. Janis, "Psychological Effects of Electric Convulsive Treatments (I. Post-Treatment Amnesia) *Journal of Nervous and Mental Diseases* 111, 5 (May 1950) 359–382.

40 Work by Ottoson helped to establish that a convulsion was necessary for the therapy to be effective. This finding provided refutation for the views that ECT worked because it was a dramatic ritual, as well as psychoanalytic ideas that ECT worked by providing external punishment and thus replacing the role of the punitive superego.

41 Borje Cronholm and Jan-Otto Ottosson, "The Experience of Memory Function after Electroconvulsive Therapy," *British Journal of Psychiatry* 109 (1963) 251–258.

42 Emil N. Zamora and Rudolf Kaelbling, "Memory and Electroconvulsive Therapy," *American Journal of Psychiatry* 122 (1965) 546–554; David J. Impastato and William Karliner, "Control of Memory Impairment in EST by Unilateral Stimulation of the Non-Dominant Hemisphere," *Diseases of the Nervous System* XXVII, 3 (March 1966) 183–188.

43 Sackeim et al., "Cognitive Effects of Electroconvulsive Therapy in Community Settings." The claim that unilateral placement had milder adverse effects without loss of efficacy is not entirely new; see, for example, D. Cronin, P. Bodley, and L. Potts, "Unilateral and Bilateral ECT: A Study of Memory Disturbance and Relief from Depression," *Journal of Neurology, Neurosurgery, and Psychiatry* 33 (1970) 705–713.

44 Moyra Williams, "Memory Disorders Associated with Electroconvulsive Therapy," in C. W. M. Whitty and O. L. Zangwill, eds., *Amnesia* (London: Butterworths, 1966). See also Rhea L. Dornbush, "Memory and Induced ECT Convulsions," *Seminars in Psychiatry* 4, 1 (February 1972) 47–54; Larry R. Squire and Patricia L. Miller, "Diminution of Anterograde Amnesia following Electroconvulsive Therapy," *British Journal of Psychiatry* 125 (1974) 490–495; and Edgar Miller, "The Effect of ECT on Memory and Learning," *British Journal of Medical Psychology* 43, 57 (1970) 57–62, which confirmed that ECT produces memory disturbances, but expressed skepticism about permanent losses.

45 See, for example, William W. K. Zung, Judith Rogers, and Arnold Krugman, "Effect of Electroconvulsive Therapy on Memory in Depressive Disorders," in Joseph Wortis, ed., *Recent Advances in Biological Psychiatry* (New York: Plenum Press, 1968).

46 C. G. Costello, G. P. Belton, J. C. Abra, and B. E. Dunn, "The Amnesic and Therapeutic Effects of Bilateral and Unilateral ECT," *British Journal of Psychiatry* 116 (1970) 69–78.

47 Costello et al., "Amnesic and Therapeutic Effects," 76.

48 Costello et al., "Amnesic and Therapeutic Effects," 77.

49 Borje Cronholm, "Post-ECT Amnesias," in George A. Talland and Nancy C. Waugh, eds., *The Pathology of Memory* (New York: Academic Press, 1969).

50 Rhea L. Dornbush, "Memory and Induced ECT Convulsions." There was some speculation in the ECT research community at this time that unilateral placement was more dangerous because a more posterior placement affected the temporal lobes of the brain.

51 Robert G. Harper and Arthur N. Wiens, "Electroconvulsive Therapy and Memory," *The Journal of Nervous and Mental Disease* 161, 4 (1975) 245–254.

52 Harper and Wiens, "Electroconvulsive Therapy and Memory," 251.

53 Larry R. Squire, Pamela C. Slater, and Patricia L. Miller, "Retrograde Amnesia and Bilateral Electroconvulsive Therapy," *Archives of General Psychiatry* 38 (January 1981) 89–95; W. F. Daniel and H. F. Crovitz, "Acute Memory Impairment following Electroconvulsive Therapy 2. Effects of Electrode Placement," *Acta Psychiatrica Scandinavica* 67 (1983) 57–68.

54 Wallace Shellenberger, Marvin J. Miller, Iver F. Small, Victor Milstein, and James Stout, "Follow-up Study of Memory Deficits After ECT," *Canadian Journal of Psychiatry* 217 (June 1982) 325–329. The authors failed to show less hypothesized adverse effect with brief pulse. But Daniel and Crovitz asserted in "Acute Memory Impairment following Electroconvulsive Therapy" that most studies had supported this.

55 These included Larry R. Squire and Patricia L. Miller, "Diminution of Anterograde Amnesia following Electroconvulsive Therapy," *British Journal of Psychiatry* 125 (1974) 490–495; Larry R. Squire, Pamela C. Slater, and Paul M. Chace, "Retrograde Amnesia: Temporal Gradient in Very Long-Term Memory following Electroconvulsive Therapy," *Science* New Series 187, 4171 (January 10, 1975) 77–79; Larry R. Squire, Pamela C. Slater, and Paul M. Chace, "Anterograde Amnesia following Electroconvulsive Therapy: No Evidence for State-Dependent Learning," *Behavioral Biology* 17 (1976) 31–41; Larry R. Squire, C. Douglas Wetzel, and Pamela C. Slater, "Memory Complaint After Electroconvulsive Therapy: Assessment with a New Self-Rating Instrument," *Biological Psychiatry* 14, 5 (October 1979) 791–801; Larry R. Squire, Pamela C. Slater, and Patricia L. Miller, "Retrograde Amnesia and Bilateral Electroconvulsive Therapy," *Archives of General Psychiatry* 38 (January 1981) 89–95; and Larry R. Squire and Pamela C. Slater, "Electroconvulsive Therapy and Complaints of Memory Dysfunction: A Prospective Three-Year Follow-up Study," *British Journal of Psychiatry* 142 (1983) 1–8.

56 Squire, Slater, and Chace, "Retrograde Amnesia: Temporal Gradient in Very Long-Term Memory following Electroconvulsive Therapy." This finding was consonant with the classic finding named Ribot's Law, after the French psychologist Theodule Ribot who formulated it, that amnesia caused by brain injury or illness will affect remote memories least.

57 Squire and Miller, "Diminution of Anterograde Amnesia following Electroconvulsive Therapy"; Larry R. Squire, C. Douglas Wetzel, and Pamela C. Slater, "Memory Complaint After Electroconvulsive Therapy: Assessment with a New Self-Rating Instrument," *Biological Psychiatry* 14, 5 (October 1979) 791–801; Squire, Slater, and Miller, "Retrograde Amnesia and Bilateral Electroconvulsive Therapy"; Larry R. Squire and Pamela C. Slater, "Electroconvulsive Therapy and Complaints of Memory Dysfunction: A Prospective Three-Year Follow-up Study," *British Journal of Psychiatry* 142 (1983) 1–8.

58 Squire and Slater, "Electroconvulsive Therapy and Complaints of Memory Dysfunction: A Prospective Three-Year Follow-up Study."

59 Squire, Wetzel, and Slater, "Memory Complaint after Electroconvulsive Therapy: Assessment with a New Self-Rating Instrument."

60 Squire and Slater, "Electroconvulsive Therapy and Complaints of Memory Dysfunction: A Prospective Three-Year Follow-up Study."

61 Trevor R. P. Price, "Short and Long-Term Cognitive Effects of ECT: Part 1—Effects on Memory," *Psychopharmacology Bulletin* 18, 2 (April 1982) 81–91.

62 C. P. L. Freeman and R. E. Kendell, "ECT: II: Patients Who Complain," *British Journal of Psychiatry* 137 (1980) 17–25.

63 Price, "Short and Long-Term Cognitive Effects of ECT," 86.

64 Shellenberger, Miller, Small, Milstein, and Stout, "Follow-up Study of Memory Deficits After ECT," 325.

65 Squire and Slater, "Electroconvulsive Therapy and Complaints of Memory Dysfunction: A Prospective Three-Year Follow-up Study," 1.

66 Richard D. Weiner, "Does Electroconvulsive Therapy Cause Brain Damage?" *The Behavioral and Brain Sciences* 7 (1984) 1–53.

67 This point—that psychiatric treatment is intended to work on the brain, and thus must change it in some way—was one I heard ECT researcher Sarah Lisanby make at a panel at the 2004 American Psychiatric Association meetings in New York.

68 Weiner, "Does Electroconvulsive Therapy Cause Brain Damage?" 43.

69 Helen M. Pettinati and Joanne Rosenberg, "Memory Ratings Before and After Electroconvulsive Therapy: Depression- *versus* ECT Induced," *Biological Psychiatry* 19, 4 (1984) 539–548.

70 Avraham Calev, Edna Be-Tzvi, Baruch Shapira, Heinz Drexler, Refael Carasso, and Bernard Lerer, "Distinct Memory Impairments following Electroconvulsive Therapy and Imipramine," *Psychological Medicine* 19 (1989) 111–119.

71 Alexander L. Miller, Raymond A. Faber, John P. Hatch, and Harold E. Alexander, "Factors Affecting Amnesia, Seizure Duration, and Efficacy in ECT," *American Journal of Psychiatry* 42, 6 (June 1985) 692–696.

72 Richard D. Weiner, Helen J. Rogers, Jonathan R.T. Davidson, and Larry R. Squire, "Effects of Stimulus Parameters on Cognitive Side Effects," in Sidney Malitz and Harold A. Sackeim, eds., *Electroconvulsive Therapy: Clinical and Basic Research Issues, Annals of the New York Academy of Sciences* (New York: The New York Academy of Sciences, 1986).

73 Christina Sobin, Harold A. Sackeim, Joan Prudic, D.P. Devanand, Bobba J. Moody, and Martin C. McElhiney, "Predictors of Retrograde Amnesia following ECT," *American Journal of Psychiatry* 152, 7 (July 1995) 995–1001.

74 Sarah H. Lisanby, Jill H. Maddox, Joan Prudic, D.P. Devanand, and Harold Sackeim, "The Effects of Electroconvulsive Therapy on Memory of Autobiographical and Public Events," *Archives of General Psychiatry* 57 (June 2000) 581–590.

75 See, for example, D.P. Devanand, Anil K. Verma, Fughik Tirumalasetti, and Harold A. Sackeim, "Absence of Cognitive Impairment After More than 100 Lifetime ECT Treatments," *American Journal of Psychiatry* 148, 7 (July 1991) 929–932.

76 Harold Sackeim, "Editorial: Memory and ECT: From Polarization to Reconciliation," *The Journal of ECT* 16, 2 (2001) 87–96.

77 Sackeim, "Editorial: Memory and ECT," 87, emphasis added.

78 Sackeim, 2001, 88.

79 Hirshbein, "Electroconvulsive Therapy, Memory, and Self in America."

80 Max Fink, *Electroshock: Restoring the Mind* (New York: Oxford University Press, 1999), ix.

81 Fink, *Electroshock,* 16. On the following page, Fink concedes that there are cases of permanent memory loss, but asserts that they are very rare.

82 Abrams, *Electroconvulsive Therapy.*

83 Kellner, Pritchett, Beale, and Coffey, *Handbook of ECT,* 87–90.

84 Charles Kellner, "ECT in the Media," *Psychiatric Annals* 28, 9 (September 1998) 528–529.

85 Without using precise diagnostic language, it is clear that Hemingway suffered from mental illness, including a noticeable break with reality in 1959. See Kenneth S. Lynn, *Hemingway* (Cambridge: Harvard University Press, 1987), 578–579.

86 https://medium.com/cuepoint/a-family-in-peril-lou-reed-s-sister-sets-the-record-straight-about-his-childhood-20e8399f84a3#.ypehtez3q, accessed February 18, 2016.

87 Legs McNeil and Gillian McCain, *Please Kill Me: The Uncensored Oral History of Punk* (New York: Penguin, 1996), 3.

88 McNeil and McCain, *Please Kill Me,* 3.

89 Judith Kruger, *My Fight for Sanity* (Greenwich: Crest Books, 1959).

90 Kruger, *My Fight,* 55.
91 Kruger, *My Fight,* 68.
92 Kruger, *My Fight,* 69–70.
93 Kruger, *My Fight,* 73.
94 Wolfe, *Aftershock.*
95 Wolfe, *Aftershock,* 96, emphasis in original.
96 Wolfe, *Aftershock,* 83, emphasis in original.
97 On this point, see Jesse Ballenger, *Self, Senility, and Alzheimer's Disease in Modern America: A History* (Baltimore: The Johns Hopkins University Press, 2006).
98 Wolfe, *Aftershock,* 198.
99 Charles Kellner, "Editorial: The Cognitive Effects of ECT: Bridging the Gap between Research and Clinical Practice," *Convulsive Therapy* 12, 3 (1996) 133–135.
100 Marion Milner, *The Hands of the Living God: An Account of a Psycho-analytic Treatment* (London: Virago Press, 1988, originally published 1969).
101 Milner, *The Hands of the Living God,* xxix.
102 Burton Roueché, "As Empty as Eve," *The New Yorker,* September 9, 1974, 84–100.
103 Roueché, "As Empty as Eve," 87.
104 Roueché, "As Empty as Eve," 88.
105 Roueché, "As Empty as Eve," 94.
106 Roueché, "As Empty as Eve," 96.
107 Robert M. Pirsig, *Zen and the Art of Motorcycle Maintenance: An Inquiry into Values* (New York: Bantam Books, 1974). Given how widely this book has been read, and therefore how influential it likely has been in shaping public perception of ECT, this book has been oddly neglected by historians of ECT and other somatic treatments for mental illness; I am aware of no historical account that mentions it.
108 Pirsig, *Zen and the Art of Motorcycle Maintenance,* 33. There are many similar passages in the book.
109 Andrew Solomon, *The Noonday Demon: An Atlas of Depression* (New York: Scribner, 2001).
110 Solomon, *The Noonday Demon,* 74–77. "Bill Stein" is a pseudonym Solomon assigned.
111 Solomon, *The Noonday Demon,* 75.
112 Solomon, *The Noonday Demon,* 122.
113 Solomon, *The Noonday Demon,* 162–163. Solomon also tells of the case of Angel Starkey, who had endemic memory problems due to ECT; Solomon, *The Noonday Demon,* 423.
114 Martha Manning, *Undercurrents: A Life beneath the Surface* (New York: HarperSanFrancisco, 1994).
115 Solomon, *Noon-Day Demon,* 123.
116 Manning, *Undercurrents,* 102, 109.
117 Manning, *Undercurrents,* 150.
118 Manning, *Undercurrents,* 130.
119 Donahue, "Electroconvulsive Therapy and Memory Loss," 135.
120 Donahue, "Electroconvulsive Therapy and Memory Loss," 138.
121 Donahue, "Electroconvulsive Therapy and Memory Loss," 135.
122 Anne B. Donahue, "Riding the Mental Health Pendulum: Mixed Messages in the Era of Neurobiology and Self-Help Movements," *Social Work* 45, 5 (October 2000) 427–438.
123 Andy Behrman, *Electroboy: A Memoir of Mania* (New York: Random House, 2002).

124 Andy Behrman, "Electroboy," *New York Times Magazine,* January 17, 1999.
125 Terri Cheney, *Manic: A Memoir* (New York: HarperCollins Publishers, 2008). I thank Christine Mueri for the reference.
126 Cheney, *Manic,* 168.
127 Cheney, *Manic,* 172.
128 Cheney, *Manic,* 166–167.
129 Cheney, *Manic,* 2.
130 Jonathan Cott, *On the Sea of Memory: A Journey from Forgetting to Remembering* (New York: Random House, 2005).
131 Cott, *On the Sea of Memory,* 4–8.
132 Cott, *On the Sea of Memory,* 22–23.
133 Cott, *On the Sea of Memory,* 8.
134 Carrie Fisher, *Shockaholic* (New York: Simon and Schuster, 2011).
135 Fisher, *Shockaholic,* 20.
136 Fisher, *Shockaholic,* 19.
137 Linda Andre, *Doctors of Deception: What They Don't Want You to Know about Shock Therapy* (New Brunswick: Rutgers University Press, 2009). For another recent account that is more uniformly negative, see Wendy Funk's memoir of her involuntary ECT, *What Difference Does It Make? The Journey of a Soul Survivor* (Cranbrook, British Columbia: Wild Flower Publishing, 1998).
138 There are many memoirs of antidepressant usage—I have a read a number of them and teach a course that covers many of them. I have yet to see one that laments lost memory from the treatment as a major theme.
139 Price, "Short and Long-Term Cognitive Effects of ECT."
140 I am grateful to Nick King for discussions on this point.
141 Hirshbein, "Electroconvulsive Therapy, Memory, and Self in America"; Jesse Ballenger, *Self, Senility, and Alzheimer's Disease in Modern America;* Emily Martin, *Bipolar Expeditions: Mania and Depression in American Culture* (Princeton: Princeton University Press, 2009).
142 Solomon, *Noon-Day Demon,* 286.
143 Arthur J. Barsky and Jonathan Borus, "Somatization and Medicalization in the Era of Managed Care," *Journal of the American Medical Association* 274 (1995) 1931–1934.
144 Peter Breggin, *Electroshock: Its Brain-Disabling Effects* (New York: Springer Publications, 1979).
145 Perhaps the most famous expression of this is Charlotte Perkins Gilman's novella *The Yellow Wallpaper*. The feminist historiography on this point with regard to psychiatry is mountainous, but a touchstone for me has been Elaine Showalter, *The Female Malady* (New York: Viking, 1985). For a recent study that looks at this in another realm of medicine see Wendy Kline, *Bodies of Knowledge: Sexuality: Reproduction, and Women's Health in the Second Wave* (Chicago: University of Chicago Press, 2010).

Conclusion

ECT has been controversial because of the one thing all observers have agreed upon: its power. In nearly 80 years of use, virtually no one has doubted that ECT has powerful effects on body and mind.

The power of ECT has made it a flash point in a number of proxy battles. These battles are about what we wish for, and what we fear, from medicine. They are battles over the value of invasive treatments, about the prestige of doctors and the possible risks in submitting to medical authority, about the nature and costs of medical progress, about the role of medicine as a tool of social enforcement, about the degree of risk we should accept from a psychiatric treatment, and whether in fact psychiatry is properly considered a part of medicine. They have been battles over what a person is, what the basic nature of the self is. ECT has not been unique in raising these questions. But its undeniable power has raised them with dramatic intensity.

I have sought to avoid making this book a work of advocacy for or against ECT. This is not because I think history should not be advocacy, and still less because I do not have personal opinions about ECT. My opinions, in brief, are that ECT is a valuable part of medicine's repertoire, for those who need it. I also hope that I never need it, both because I hope I am never that ill, and because it incurs risks other treatments for affective disorders do not. I also think that involuntary ECT should be especially avoided, and that ECT given with consent should come with a warning that at least some patients do experience serious permanent memory losses, and we are not really sure how many. My decision to attempt to step back and examine the structures of the controversies around ECT came, then, not from lack of opinions about it, but rather from a sense that discussions of ECT had become so locked into a for-or-against posture that they have become shackled to either/or arguments. Stepping back and historicizing the controversy itself allows us to learn more from the history of the treatment.

One way I have emphasized this is in the way we think about medical progress. Historians of medicine have battled against naïve, heroic, linear, and teleological ideas of progress for some time now. This has not been a trivial fight. Seeing progress in these terms can lead to hard practical consequences, in the quest for progress at all costs, and in the fueling of false hope and expectations of what medicine can accomplish. In psychiatry, the expectation of progress has too often led to a cycle of clinical hype, where the potential for adverse effects from treatment are noticed too slowly. We also should not be too dismissive, though, about what medical progress has meant. Medical historians have become very skilled at disrupting "progress narratives," but illness has been a central source of suffering throughout humankind's history. Medicine helped to make significant, if uneven, headway against this in industrial modernity. Psychiatry has, I believe, shared in this. We do not have, as yet, a penicillin of psychiatry. Psychiatry's repertoire of treatments to alleviate suffering is, though, substantially richer in 2016 than it was in 1916.

Innovation in non-pharmaceutical psychiatric somatic treatments has actually been modest since the 1950s. New therapies such as deep brain stimulation and transcranial magnetic stimulation are promising therapeutic effects at least comparable to ECT, with lower risk of adverse effects.[1] Some reins on enthusiasm may seem warranted, as the history of somatic treatments has shown that adverse effects are not always recognized early in a new treatment's use. But it would be equally uncritical to allow for no possibility of progress. Whatever flaws there may be in current treatments, from ECT to antidepressants and antipsychotic medications, they remain good reasons not to revive the use of insulin coma therapy. We need to be careful in touting new psychiatric treatments. We should not, though, be scornful or reflexively hostile to the idea of medical progress. Medical progress is an uneven and contested process, not a mythical or heroic inevitability, but if we abandon any notion of progress, or lament any attempts to document progress as ahistorical or quaint, we lose as much capacity for critical judgment as we do when we assume a teleological viewpoint. Within ECT practice itself there has been progress. Used as it often is now—modified, with consent, a last resort after less risky treatments are tried, and one for which we would like to find alternatives— is itself progress from an era where unmodified ECT was used often on unwilling patients.

As ECT has returned to clinical favor and relatively widespread use, there has not been an adequate reckoning with the complexity of its history. A desire to reduce the stigma surrounding ECT, and thereby promote its use among scared patients who might benefit, has led to a number of portrayals that have presented ECT as essentially harmless. It is hard, to say the least, to square this portrayal with both clinical research that documents at least some risks, and decades of significant patient complaints. It's true that the nature of the complaints change, and it is also true that many patients do not complain. There is a significant history of dismissal of complaints about ECT, though, which has not served anyone well.

It becomes clearer that ECT has not been intrinsically purely therapeutic or purely disciplinary, but became more or less one or the other depending upon how it was used. In turn, this illustrates that we do not have to make blanket judgments about whether somatic treatments, whether shock thera-pies or drugs, are inherently good or bad things. Like all medical treatments, they carry both risks and benefits.

The importance of this lesson for clinical practice is enormous.[2] There is abundant evidence that patients can benefit from both somatic treatments and talk therapies, and can often benefit from the two together. They might, of course, benefit in different ways. Many will welcome the relief from, or control of, symptoms that somatic treatments can offer, often quickly. Many will welcome the exploration of meaning and long-term benefits that dynamic therapy can offer. Many will simply want one or the other, or will want them to complement each other.

Elyn Saks's memoir of her struggle with schizophrenia is a powerful illus-tration.[3] Saks suffered for years before she found herself able to say that she in fact had an illness, and believed at first that needing medications was a sign of failure. To her, taking medications meant something was wrong with her, in a way that psychoanalysis did not. By contrast, psychoanalytic interpretation of the meaning of her thoughts was something she always found therapeutic. For other psychiatric patients, something like the oppo-site could be true—they might feel that the usefulness of a somatic treatment showed that they had a real disease, whereas plunging into memories of life events was the distasteful treatment. When Saks came to believe that she would need to be on medications for life, the new value she found in them did not lead her to discard psychoanalysis. Rather, she came to see the two modalities as working in concert. Saks's story shows that people managing symptoms of madness are often less interested in a dogmatic conception of a certain kind of science or a certain conception of personhood than they are in relief of suffering.

The rigidity with which some advocates insist that a humane or scientific psychiatry must be either somatic or talk frankly puzzles me. Mental dis-tress is layered with mystery. There are mountains of evidence to show that our inner lives spring from biological, psychological, and social sources, and we still have a very poor grasp on the extent to which these sources are even discrete, separable things. The history of psychiatry is replete with clinicians and patient advocates claiming the complete and final victory of one modality (talk or somatic) over another. Historians should not repeat this mistake. To the extent we do, we are reproducing an ideology of our object of study.

Social and cultural historians consider it a calling to recover voices, and in medical history this has meant, to a large extent, patients. This recovery is never complete, and it is likely that many patients who felt very damaged by ECT were never able to record their story, and many who felt helped never bothered to. Of the voices captured here, there is the undoubted presence of some on one extreme or the other, and also a wealth of accounts that labor to show a commingling of healing and loss. Taken together, they defy reduc-tion to easy tropes of medical abuse or miracle cure.

Notes

1 See Sarah Lisanby, ed., *Brain Stimulation in Psychiatric Treatment* (Washington, D.C.: American Psychiatric Publishing Inc., 2004).
2 This paragraph and the two that follow it are adapted from my chapter "Somatic Treatments," in Greg Eghigian, ed., *The Routledge History of Madness* (forthcoming).
3 Elyn R. Saks, *The Center Cannot Hold: My Journey through Madness* (New York: Hachette Books, 2007).

Bibliography

Newspaper and Magazine Articles

Behrman, Andy. "Electroboy," *New York Times Magazine,* January 17, 1999.

Brody, Jane E. "Shock Therapy Loses Some of Its Shock Value," *New York Times,* September 19, 2006.

Crews, Frederick. "Talking Back to Prozac," *The New York Review of Books,* December 6, 2007.

Farnsworth, Clyde. "Canada Will Pay 50's Test Victims," *New York Times,* November 19, 1992.

Makari, George. "Notes from Psychiatry's Battle Lines," *New York Times,* February 23, 2016.

McCoubrey, Carmel. "Dr. Gerard Chrzanowski, Innovative Psychoanalyst, Dies at 87," *New York Times,* November 12, 2000.

Pace, Eric. "Lothar Kalinowsky, A Psychiatrist, 92; Used Electroshocks," *New York Times,* June 30, 1992.

Roueché, Burton. "As Empty as Eve," *The New Yorker,* September 9, 1974, 84–100.

Saxon, Wolfgang. "L. Bryce Boyer," *New York Times,* August 26, 2000.

Treaster, Joseph B. "Army Discloses Man Died in Drug Test It Sponsored," *New York Times,* August 13, 1975.

Ward, Mary Jane. "Out of the Dark Ages," *Woman's Home Companion,* August, 1946.

Dissertation

Gambino, Matthew Joseph. *Mental Health and Ideals of Citizenship: Patient Care at St. Elizabeth's Hospital in Washington D.C., 1903–1962,* Ph. D. dissertation, University of Illinois at Urbana-Champaign, 2010.

Journal Articles

Abrams, Richard. "Lothar Kalinowsky, M. D., 1899–1992," *Convulsive Therapy* 8, 3 (1992) 218–220.

Almansi, Renato and David J. Impastato, "Electrically Induced Convulsions in the Treatment of Mental Diseases," *New York State Journal of Medicine* 40, 17 (September 1, 1940) 1315.

Alper, Thelma. "An Electric Shock Patient Tells His Story," *Journal of Abnormal and Social Psychology* 43 (1944) 201–210.

Alverno, Luca. "The Origins of Electroconvulsive Therapy," *Wisconsin Medical Journal* (February 1990) 54–56.

Barsky, Arthur J. and Jonathan Borus, "Somatization and Medicalization in the Era of Managed Care," *Journal of the American Medical Association* 274 (1995) 1931–1934.

Bateman, J. Fremont and H. Warren Dunham, "The State Mental Hospital as a Specialized Community Experience," *American Journal of Psychiatry* 105, 6 (December 1948) 445–448.

Bennett, A. E. "Preventing Traumatic Complications in Convulsive Shock Therapy by Curare," *Journal of the American Medical Association* 114 (1940) 322–324.

———. "Curare: A Preventive of Traumatic Complications in Convulsive Shock Therapy," *American Journal of Psychiatry* 97 (1941) 1040–1060.

Beskow, Jan and Tore Hallstrom, "In Honour of Jan-Otto Ottoson," *Acta Psychiatrica Scandinavia* (1991) 399–400.

Boyer, L. Bryce. "Fantasies Concerning Convulsive Therapy," *Psychoanalytic Review* 39 (1952) 252–270.

Brill, H. "Paul Hoch: Administrator," *Comprehensive Psychiatry* 6, 2 (April 1965) 67–70.

Brody, M. B. "Prolonged Memory Defects following Electro-Therapy," *Journal of Mental Science* 90, 380 (July 1944) 777–779.

Burnham, John C. "Why Sociologists Abandoned the Sick Role Concept," *History of the Human Sciences* 27, 1 (2014) 70–87.

Burns, G. E. "The Scientific Origins of Electroconvulsive Therapy: A Conceptual History," *History of Psychiatry* viii (1997) 105–119.

Bustin, Julian, Mark J. Rapoport, Murali Krishna, Daniel Matusevich, Carlos Finkelsztein, Sergio Strejilevich, and David Anderson, "Are Patients' Attitudes towards and Knowledge of Electroconvulsive Therapy Transcultural? A Multi-National Pilot Study," *International Journal of Geriatric Psychiatry* 23 (2008) 497–503.

Calev, Abraham, Edna Be-Tzvi, Baruch Shapira, Heinz Drexler, Refael Carasso, and Bernard Lerer, "Distinct Memory Impairments following Electroconvulsive Therapy and Imipramine," *Psychological Medicine* 19 (1989) 111–119.

Cameron, D. Ewen. "The Current Transition in the Conception of Science," *Science,* new series 107, 2787 (May 28, 1948) 553–558.

Cameron, D. Ewen, Leonard Levy, Thomas Ban, and Leonard Rubenstein, "Automation of Psychotherapy," *Comprehensive Psychiatry* 5, 1 (February 1964) 1–14.

Codr, Dwight. "Arresting Monstrosity: Polio, Frankenstein, and the Horror Film," *PMLA* (March 2014) 171–187.

Costello, C. G., G. P. Belton, J. C. Abra, and B. E. Dunn, "The Amnesic and Therapeutic Effects of Bilateral and Unilateral ECT," *British Journal of Psychiatry* 116 (1970) 69–78.

Cronholm Borje and Jan-Otto Ottosson, "The Experience of Memory Function after Electroconvulsive Therapy," *British Journal of Psychiatry* 109 (1963) 251–258.

Cronin, D., P. Bodley, and L. Potts, "Unilateral and Bilateral ECT: A Study of Memory Disturbance and Relief from Depression," *Journal of Neurology, Neurosurgery, and Psychiatry* 33 (1970) 705–713.

Daniel, W. F. and H. F. Crovitz, "Acute Memory Impairment following Electroconvulsive Therapy 2: Effects of Electrode Placement," *Acta Psychiatrica Scandinavica* 67 (1983) 57–68.

Devanand, D.P., Anil K. Verma, Fughik Tirumalasetti, and Harold A. Sackeim, "Absence of Cognitive Impairment after More than 100 Lifetime ECT Treatments," *American Journal of Psychiatry* 148, 7 (July 1991) 929–932.

Donahue, Anne B. "Electroconvulsive Therapy and Memory Loss: A Personal Journey," *The Journal of ECT* 16, 2 (2000) 133–143.

Dornbush, Rhea L. "Memory and Induced ECT Convulsions," *Seminars in Psychiatry* 4, 1 (February 1972) 47–54, and Larry R. Squire and Patricia L. Miller, "Diminution of Anterograde Amnesia following Electroconvulsive Therapy," *British Journal of Psychiatry* 125 (1974) 490–495.

Doroshow, D.B. "Performing a Cure for Schizophrenia: Insulin Coma Therapy on the Wards," *Journal of the History of Medicine and Allied Sciences* 62, 2 (2007) 213–243.

Endler, Norman S. "The Origins of Electroconvulsive Therapy (ECT)," *Convulsive Therapy* 4, 1 (1988) 5–23.

Etkin, Nina. "'Side Effects': Cultural Constructions and Reinterpretations of Western Pharmaceuticals," *Medical Anthropology Quarterly* 6, 2 (1992) 99–113.

Finger, Stanley. "Medical Electricity and Madness in the 18th Century," *Perspectives in Biology and Medicine* 49, 3 (Summer 2006) 330–345.

Finger, Stanley and Franklin Zaromb, "Benjamin Franklin and Shock-Induced Amnesia," *American Psychologist* 61, 3 (April 2006) 240–248.

Fink, Max. "What Is an Adequate Treatment in Convulsive Therapy?" *Acta Psychiatrica Scandinavia* 84 (1991) 424–427.

Fink, Max and Charles Kellner, "The Perplexing History of ECT in Three Books," *Psychiatric Times*, August 12, 2010.

Freedman, Alfred. "Lothar Kalinowsky, M.D., 1899–1992," *Comprehensive Psychiatry* 33, 6 (November/December 1992) 357–358.

Freeman, C.P.L. and R.E. Kendell, "ECT: II: Patients Who Complain," *British Journal of Psychiatry* 137 (1980) 17–25.

Freyman, F.A. "Tribute to Paul Hoch," *Comprehensive Psychiatry* 6, 2 (April 1965) 67–70.

Gazdag, Gabor, Max Fink, Gabor S. Ungvari, and Edward Shorter, "Laszlo Meduna's Immigration to the United States in 1939," *Journal of ECT* 26, 2 (June 2010) 79–81.

Gonda, Victor. "Treatment of Mental Disorders with Electrically Induced Convulsions," *Diseases of the Nervous System* 2, 844 (March 1941) 84–92.

Gottesfeld, Ben H. and Calvin Barker, "An Interpretive Study of Subjective Response to Electric Shock Therapy," *Digest of Neurology and Psychiatry* 14, 642 (1946) 642–648.

Greenberg, Robert M. and Charles H. Kellner, "Electroconvulsive Therapy: A Selected Review," *American Journal of Geriatric Psychiatry* 13, 4 (April 2005) 268–281.

Grinker, Roy R. and Helen V. McLean, "The Course of a Depression Treated by Psychotherapy and Metrazol," *Psychosomatic Medicine* 2, 2 (April 1940) 119–138.

Grob, Gerald. "The Attack of Psychiatric Legitimacy in the 1960s: Rhetoric and Reality," *Journal of the History of the Behavioral Sciences* 47, 4 (2011) 398–416.

Harper, Robert G. and Arthur N. Wiens, "Electroconvulsive Therapy and Memory," *The Journal of Nervous and Mental Disease* 161, 4 (1975) 245–254.

Herzig, Rebecca. "Subjected to the Current: Batteries, Bodies, and the Early History of Electrification in the United States," *Journal of Social History* 41 (Summer 2008) 867–885.

Hilton, Claire. "An Exploration of the Patient's Experience of Electro-convulsive Therapy in Mid-twentieth Century Creative Literature: A Historical Study with Implications for Practice Today," *Journal of Affective Disorders* 97 (2007) 5–12.

Hirshbein, Laura. "Electroconvulsive Therapy, Memory, and Self in America," *Journal of the History of the Neurosciences: Basic and Clinical Perspectives* 21, 2 (2012) 147–169.

Holland, C.G. "The Complaint of 'Forgetting' following Electroshock," *Virginia Medical Monthly* (May 1950) 221–226.

Impastato, David J. "The Story of the First Electroshock Treatment," *American Journal of Psychiatry* 116 (1959–60) 1112–1114.

Impastato, David J. and William Karliner, "Control of Memory Impairment in EST by Unilateral Stimulation of the Non-Dominant Hemisphere," *Diseases of the Nervous System* XXVII, 3 (March 1966) 183–188.

Janis, Irving L. "Psychological Effects of Electric Convulsive Treatments (I. Post-Treatment Amnesia)," *Journal of Nervous and Mental Diseases* 111, 5 (May 1950) 359–382.

Kalinowsky, Lothar. "Electric-Convulsion Therapy in Schizophrenia," *The Lancet* (December 9, 1939) 1232–1233.

Kalinowsky, L. and S. Eugene Barrera, "Electric Convulsion Therapy in Mental Disorders," *Psychiatric Quarterly* 14, 719 (October 1940) 719–730.

Kellner, Charles. "Editorial: The Cognitive Effects of ECT: Bridging the Gap between Research and Clinical Practice," *Convulsive Therapy* 12, 3 (1996) 133–135.

———. "ECT in the Media," *Psychiatric Annals* 28, 9 (September 1998) 528–529.

Kennedy, Foster. "Commentary," *Journal of Nervous and Mental Diseases* 104 (July 1946) 320.

Kimball, Frank. "Hope for Tired Minds," *Hygeia* (December 1946) 906–901 & 946 and (January 1947) 36–37 & 66–69.

Kramer, Peter D. *Listening to Prozac* (New York: Viking Press, 1993).

Lebensohn, Zigmond M. "The History of Electroconvulsive Therapy and Its Place in American Psychiatry: A Personal Memoir," *Comprehensive Psychiatry* 40, 3 (May/June 1999) 173–181.

Levy, Norman and Roy Grinker, "Psychological Observations in Affective Psychoses Treated with Combined Convulsive Shock and Psychotherapy," *The Journal of Nervous and Mental Disease* 97, 6 (June 1943) 623.

Lewis, Nolan D.C. "The Present Status of Shock Therapy of Mental Disorders," *Bulletin of the New York Academy of Medicine* (April 1943) 227–243.

Liebman, Samuel. "Homosexuality, Transvestism, and Psychosis: Study of a Case Treated with Electroshock," *Journal of Nervous and Mental Disease* 99 (1949) 945–958.

Lisanby, Sarah H., Jill H. Maddox, Joan Prudic, D.P. Devanand, and Harold Sackeim, "The Effects of Electroconvulsive Therapy on Memory of Autobiographical and Public Events," *Archives of General Psychiatry* 57 (June 2000) 581–590.

Malitz, Sydney. "Paul Hoch, 1902–1964," *American Journal of Psychiatry* 153, 10 (October 1996) 1339.

Malzberg, Benjamin. "The Outcome of Electric Shock Therapy in the New York Civil State Hospitals," *Psychiatric Quarterly* 17 (1943) 154–163.

Miller, Alexander L., Raymond A. Faber, John P. Hatch, and Harold E. Alexander, "Factors Affecting Amnesia, Seizure Duration, and Efficacy in ECT," *American Journal of Psychiatry* 42, 6 (June 1985) 692–696.

Miller, Edgar. "The Effect of ECT on Memory and Learning," *British Journal of Medical Psychology* 43, 57 (1970) 57–62.

Millet, John A. P. and Eric P. Mosse, "On Certain Psychological Aspects of Electroshock Therapy," *Psychosomatic Medicine* 6, 3 (1944) 226–236. See especially 226–236.

Mosse, Eric P. "Electroshock and Personality Structure," *Journal of Nervous and Mental Diseases* 104 (July 1946) 296–302.

Myerson, Abraham, Louis Feldman, and Isadore Green, "Experience with Electric Shock Therapy in Mental Disease," *New England Journal of Medicine* 224 (1941) 1081–1085.

Neymann, Clarence. "Some Thoughts about Shock Therapy," *Archives of Physical Therapy* 24, 660 (November 1943) 660–663.

Norton, Alan. "In My Own Time: Depression," *British Medical Journal* 2 (1979) 429–430.

Ottoson, J. O. "Experimental Studies of the Mode of Action of Electroconvulsive Therapy," *Acta Psychiatrica Neurologica Scandinavia Supplement* 145 (1960) 1–141.

———. "Seizure Characteristics and Therapeutic Efficiency in Electroconvulsive Therapy: An Analysis of the Antidepressive Efficiency of Grand Mal and Lidocaine-Modified Seizures," *Journal of Nervous and Mental Diseases* 135 (1962) 239–251.

Owensby, Newdigate M. "Homosexuality and Lesbianism Treated with Metrazol: A Preliminary Report," *Journal of Nervous and Mental Diseases* 92 (July 1940) 65–66.

Passione, Roberta. "Italian Psychiatry in an International Context: Ugo Cerletti and the Case of Electroshock," *History of Psychiatry* 15, 1 (March 2004) 83–104.

Pettinati, Helen M. and Joanne Rosenberg, "Memory Ratings before and after Electroconvulsive Therapy: Depression-versus ECT Induced," *Biological Psychiatry* 19, 4 (1984) 539–548.

Pickersgill, Martin. "From Psyche to Soma? Changing Accounts of Antisocial Personality Disorders in the *American Journal of Psychiatry*," *History of Psychiatry* 21, 3 (2010) 294–311.

Porter, Roy. "The Patient's View: Doing Medical History from Below," *Theory and Society* 14, 2 (March 1985) 175–198.

Price, Trevor R. P. "Short and Long-Term Cognitive Effects of ECT: Part 1—Effects on Memory," *Psychopharmacology Bulletin* 18, 2 (April 1982) 81–91.

Prudic, Joan, Shoshana Peyser, and Harold A. Sackeim, "Subjective Memory Complaints: A Review of Patient Self-Assessment of Memory after Electroconvulsive Therapy," *The Journal of ECT* 16, 2 (2000) 121–132.

Pulver, Sydney. "The First Electroconvulsive Treatment Given in the United States," *American Journal of Psychiatry* 117 (1960–61) 845–846.

———. "Regulation of Electroconvulsive Therapy," *Michigan Law Review* 75 (1976–1977) 363–412.

Rickles, N. K. and Charles G. Polan, "Causes of Failure in Treatment with Electric Shock: Analysis of Thirty-Eight Cases," *Archives of Neurology and Psychiatry* 59 (1948) 337–346.

Rosenhan, D. L. "On Being Sane in Insane Places." *Science* 179, 70 (January 1973) 250–258.

Russell, R. J., L. G. M. Page, and R. L. Jillett, "Intensified Electroconvulsant Therapy: Review of Five Years' Experience," *The Lancet* 262, 5 (December 1953) 1177–1179.

Sackeim, Harold. "Editorial: Memory and ECT: From Polarization to Reconciliation," *The Journal of ECT* 16, 2 (2001) 87–96.

Sackeim, Harold A., Joan Prudic, Rice Fuller, John Keilp, Philip W. Lavori, and Mark Olfson, "The Cognitive Effects of Electroconvulsive Therapy in Community Settings," *Neuropsychopharmacology* 32 (2007) 244–254.

Sadowsky, Jonathan. "Review of Timothy Kneeland and Carole Warren," *Pushbutton Psychiatry, the Bulletin of the History of Medicine* 77 (2003) 471–472.

———. "Beyond the Metaphor of the Pendulum: Electroconvulsive Therapy, Psychoanalysis, and the Styles of American Psychiatry," *The Journal of the History of Medicine and Allied Sciences* 61 (January 2006) 1–25.

———. "Review of Thomas Szasz, Coercion as Cure: A Critical History of Psychiatry," *Bulletin of the History of Medicine* 83, 4 (Winter 2009) 797–798.

Scull, Andrew. "Psychiatry and Social Control in the Nineteenth and Twentieth Century," *History of Psychiatry* 2 (June 1991) 149–169.

———. "Somatic Treatments and the Historiography of Psychiatry," *History of Psychiatry* V (1994) 1–12.

Shellenberger, Wallace, Marvin J. Miller, Iver F. Small, Victor Milstein, and James Stout, "Follow-up Study of Memory Deficits after ECT," *Canadian Journal of Psychiatry* 217 (June 1982) 325–329.

Sherman, Irene and John Mergener, "The Effect of Convulsive Treatment on Memory," *American Journal of Psychiatry* 98 (November 1941) 402–403.

Sobin, Christina, Harold A. Sackeim, Joan Prudic, D. P. Devanand, Bobba J. Moody, and Martin C. McElhiney, "Predictors of Retrograde Amnesia following ECT," *American Journal of Psychiatry* 152, 7 (July 1995) 995–1001.

Squire, Larry R., C. Douglas Wetzel, and Pamela C. Slater, "Memory Complaint after Electroconvulsive Therapy: Assessment with a New Self-Rating Instrument," *Biological Psychiatry* 14, 5 (October 1979) 791–801.

Squire, Larry R. and Pamela C. Slater, "Electroconvulsive Therapy and Complaints of Memory Dysfunction: A Prospective Three-Year Follow-up Study," *British Journal of Psychiatry* 142 (1983) 1–8.

Squire, Larry R., Pamela C. Slater, and Patricia L. Miller, "Retrograde Amnesia and Bilateral Electroconvulsive Therapy," *Archives of General Psychiatry* 38 (January 1981) 89–95.

Squire, Larry R., Pamela C. Slater, and Paul M. Chace, "Retrograde Amnesia: Temporal Gradient in Very Long-Term Memory following Electroconvulsive Therapy," *Science,* new series 187, 4171 (January 10, 1975) 77–79.

Squire, Larry R., Pamela C. Slater, and Paul M. Chace, "Anterograde Amnesia following Electroconvulsive Therapy: No Evidence for State-Dependent Learning," *Behavioral Biology* 17 (1976) 31–41.

Squire, Larry R. and Patricia L. Miller, "Diminution of Anterograde Amnesia following Electroconvulsive Therapy," *British Journal of Psychiatry* 125 (1974) 490–495.

Stieper, Donald R., Meyer Williams, and Carl P. Duncan, "Changes in Impersonal and Personal Memory following Electro-Convulsive Therapy," *Journal of Clinical Psychology* VII, 4 (October 1951) 361–366.

Thompson, George N. "Electroshock and other Therapeutic Considerations in Sexual Psychopathy," *Journal of Nervous and Mental Disease* 109 (1949) 531–539.

UK ECT Review Group, "Efficacy and Safety of Electroconvulsive Therapy in Depressive Disorders: A Systematic Review and Meta-Analysis," *The Lancet* 361 (March 8, 2003) 799–808.

Weigert, Edith Vowinckel. "Psychoanalytical Notes on Sleep and Convulsion Treatment in Functional Psychoses," *Psychiatry* 3 (1940) 189–209.

Weiner, Richard D. "Does Electroconvulsive Therapy Cause Brain Damage?" *The Behavioral and Brain Sciences* 7 (1984) 1–53.

Wortis, Joseph. "Remembering Paul Hoch," *Biological Psychiatry* 35 (1994) 901–902.

Zamora, Emil N. and Rudolf Kaelbling, "Memory and Electroconvulsive Therapy," *American Journal of Psychiatry* 122 (1965) 546–554.

Zilboorg, Gregory. "The Fundamental Conflict with Psychoanalysis," *International Journal of Psychoanalysis* 20 (1939) 480–492.

Zubin, Joseph. "Paul H. Hoch's Contribution to the American Psychopathological Association," *Comprehensive Psychiatry* 6, 2 (April 1965) 74–77.

Books

Abrams, Richard. *Electroconvulsive Therapy* (4th edition, Oxford: Oxford University Press, 2002).

Adair, Nancy and Casey Adair, *Word Is Out: Stories of Some of Our Lives* (New York: Dell Publishing Co., 1978).

Andre, Linda. *Doctors of Deception: What They Don't Want You to Know about Shock Therapy* (New Brunswick: Rutgers University Press, 2009).

Arikha, Noga. *Passions and Tempers: A History of the Humours* (New York: Harper Perennial, 2007).

Auden, W. H. *Another Time: Poems* (London: Faber & Faber, 1940).

Baldwin, Steve and Melissa Oxlad, *Electroshock and Minors: A Fifty-Year Review* (Westport: Greenwood Press, 2000).

Ballenger, Jesse. *Self, Senility, and Alzheimer's Disease in Modern America: A History* (Baltimore: The Johns Hopkins University Press, 2006).

Barnes, Mary and Joseph Berke, *Mary Barnes: Two Accounts of a Journey through Madness* (New York: Harcourt Brace Jovanovich, 1971).

Bayer, Ronald. *Homosexuality and American Psychiatry* (Princeton: Princeton University Press, 1987).

Beam, Alex. *Gracefully Insane: The Rise and Fall of America's Premier Mental Hospital* (New York: PublicAffairs, 2001).

Behrman, Andy. *Electroboy: A Memoir of Mania* (New York: Random House, 2002).

Belknap, Ivan. *Human Problems of a State Mental Hospital* (New York: McGraw-Hill Book Company, 1956).

Berke, Joseph. *I Haven't Had to Go Mad Here* (Harmondsworth: Penguin Books, 1979, originally published as *Butterfly Man*, 1977).

Bertucci, Paola and Giulano Pancaldi, *Electric Bodies: Episodes in the History of Medical Electricity* (Bologna: Universita di Bologna, 2001).

Braslow, Joel. *Mental Ills and Bodily Cures: Psychiatric Treatment in the First Half of the Twentieth Century* (Berkeley: University of California, 1997).

Breggin, Peter. *Electroshock: Its Brain-Disabling Effects* (New York: Springer Publications, 1979).

Breggin, Peter. *Toxic Psychiatry: Why Therapy, Empathy, and Love Must Replace the Drugs, Electroshock, and Biochemical Theories* (New York: St. Martin's Griffin, 1994).

Bud, Robert. *Penicillin: Triumph and Tragedy* (Oxford: Oxford University Press, 2007).

Chauncey, George. *Gay New York: Gender, Urban Culture, and the Making of the Gay Male World, 1890–1940* (New York: Basic Books, 1994).

Cheney, Terri. *Manic: A Memoir* (New York: HarperCollins Publishers, 2008).

Clay, John. *R. D. Laing: A Divided Self* (London: Hodder and Stoughton, 1996).

Coffey, C. Edward. *The Clinical Science of Electro-Convulsive Therapy* (Washington, D.C.: American Psychiatric Press, Inc., 1993).

Collins, Anne. *In the Sleep Room: The Story of the CIA Brainwashing Experiments in Canada* (2nd edition, Toronto: Key Porter Books Limited, 1997, originally published 1988).

Conrad, Peter. *The Medicalization of Society: On the Transformation of Human Conditions into Treatable Diseases* (Baltimore: The Johns Hopkins University Press, 2007).

Cooter, Roger and John Pickstone eds., *Companion to Medicine in the Twentieth Century* (London: Routledge, 2003).

Cott, Jonathan. *On the Sea of Memory: A Journey from Forgetting to Remembering* (New York: Random House, 2005).

Cranford, Peter G. *But for the Grace of God: The Inside Story of the World's Largest Insane Asylum* (Augusta: Great Pyramid Press, 1981).

Csordas, Thomas. *The Sacred Self: A Cultural Phenomenology of Charismatic Healing* (Berkeley: University of California Press, 1994).

Davis-Floyd, Robbie E. *Birth as an American Rite of Passage* (2nd edition, Berkeley: University of California Press, 2003).

de la Pena, Carolyn Thomas. *The Body Electric: How Strange Machines Built the Modern American* (New York: New York University Press, 2003).

D'Emilio, John. *Lost Prophet: The Life and Times of Bayard Rustin* (New York: The Free Press, 2003).

Dowbiggin, Ian. *The Quest for Mental Health* (Cambridge: Cambridge University Press, 2011).

Duberman, Martin. *Cures: A Gay Man's Odyssey* (Cambridge, MA: Westview Press, 2002, originally published 1992).

Duffin, Jacalyn. *History of Medicine: A Scandalously Short Introduction* (Toronto: University of Toronto Press, 1999).

Dukakis, Kitty and Larry Tye, *Shock: The Healing Power of Electroconvulsive Therapy* (New York: Penguin, 2006).

Dyck, Erica. *Psychedelic Psychiatry: LSD from Clinic to Campus* (Baltimore: The Johns Hopkins University Press, 2008).

Ellison, Ralph. *Invisible Man* (New York: Vintage, 1990, originally published 1947).

Endler, Norman. *Holiday of Darkness: A Psychologist's Personal Journey Out of His Depression* (Toronto: John Wiley & Sons, Inc., 1982).

Fanon, Frantz. *The Wretched of the Earth* (New York: Grove Press, 1963).

———. *A Dying Colonialism* (New York: Grove Press, 1965).

Feldman, Gene and Max Gartenberg eds., *The Beat Generation and the Angry Young Men* (New York: The Citadel Press, 1958).

Fenichel, Otto. *The Psychoanalytic Theory of Neurosis* (New York: W. W. Norton, 1945).

Fink, Max. *Electroshock: Restoring the Mind* (New York: Oxford University Press, 1999).

Fink, Max. ed. *Psychobiology of Convulsive Therapy* (New York: V. H. Winston & Sons, 1974).

Fisher, Carrie. *Shockaholic* (New York: Simon and Schuster, 2011).

Frank, Leonard Roy. *The History of Shock Treatment* (San Francisco: Leonard Roy Frank, 1978).

Freeman, Hugh and German E. Berrios, *150 Years of British Psychiatry, Volume II: The Aftermath* (London: The Athlone Press, 1996).

Freud, Sigmund. *The Standard Edition of the Complete Psychological Works of Sigmund Freud* (James Strachey, trans., London: Hogarth Press, 1953–1974).

Funk, Wendy. *What Difference Does It Make? The Journey of a Soul Survivor* (Cranbrook, British Columbia: Wild Flower Publishing, 1998).

Gabbard, Glen. *The Psychology of the Sopranos: Love, Death, Desire and Betrayal in America's Favorite Gangster Family* (New York: Basic Books, 2002).

Gauld, Alan. *Electrotherapy in the United States* (Minneapolis: The Company, 1977).

Gelman, Sheldon. *Medicating Schizophrenia: A History* (New Brunswick: Rutgers University Press, 1999).

Gillmor, Don. *I Swear by Apollo: Dr. Ewen Cameron and the CIA-Brainwashing Experiments* (Montreal: Eden Press, 1987).

Ginsberg, Allen. "Howl," *Collected Poems, 1947–1980* (New York: Harper and Row, 1980).

Goffman, Erving. *Asylums Essays on the Social Situation of Mental Patients and Other Inmates* (Garden City: Anchor Books, 1961).

Grimes, John Maurice. *When Minds Go Wrong: A Simple Story of the Mentally Ill—Past, Present, and Future* (Chicago: Published by the Author, 1949).

Hale, Nathan. *Freud and the Americans: The Beginnings of Psychoanalysis in the United States, 1876–1917* (New York: Oxford University Press, 1971).

Hansen, Bert. *Picturing Medical Progress from Pasteur to Polio: A History of Mass Media Images and Popular Attitudes in America* (New Brunswick: Rutgers University Press, 2009).

Hart, Gary Warren. *Right from the Start: A Chronicle of the McGovern Campaign* (New York: Quadrangle/The New York Times Book Company, 1973).

Healy, David. *The Creation of Psychopharmacology* (Cambridge: Harvard University Press, 1992).

———. *The Anti-Depressant Era* (Cambridge: Harvard University Press, 1997).

———. *Let Them Eat Prozac* (New York: New York University Press, 2004).

Hirsch, Sherry, Joe Kennedy Adams, Leonard Roy Frank, Wade Hudson, Richard Keene, Gail Krawitz-Keene, David Rochman, and Robert Roth eds., *Madness Network News Reader* (San Francisco: Glide Publications, 1974).

Hirshbein, Lauta. *American Melancholy* (New Brunswick: Rutgers University Press, 2009).

Hobson, J. Allan and Jonathan A. Leonard, *Out of Its Mind: Psychiatry in Crisis* (Cambridge, MA: Perseus Publishing, 2001).

Hornstein, Gail. *Agnes's Jacket: A Psychologist's Search for the Meanings of Madness* (New York: Rodale Books, 2009).

Horwitz, Allen. *The Logic of Social Control* (New York: Plenum Press, 1990).

Hughes, Thomas P. *Networks of Power: Electrification in Western Society, 1880–1930* (Baltimore: The Johns Hopkins University Press, 1983).

Jacyna, L. Stephen and Stephen T. Casper, *The Neurological Patient in History* (Rochester: University of Rochester Press, 2012).

Jessner, Lucie and V. Gerard Ryan, *Shock Treatment in Psychiatry: A Manual* (New York: Grune and Stratton, 1941).

Johnson, David K. *Lavender Scare: The Cold War Persecution of Gays and Lesbians in the Federal Government* (Chicago: University of Chicago Press, 2006).

Johnson, Jenell. *American Lobotomy: A Rhetorical History* (Ann Arbor: University of Michigan Press, 2014).

Kalinowsky, Lothar B. and Paul H. Hoch, *Shock Treatments and Other Somatic Procedures in Psychiatry* (New York: Grune and Stratton, 1946).

Katz, Jonathan. *Gay American History: Lesbians and Gay Men in the U.S.A.* (New York: Thomas Y. Crowell, 1976).

Kellner, Charles H., John T. Pritchett, Mark D. Beale, and Edward C. Coffey, *Handbook of ECT* (Washington, D.C.: American Psychiatric Press, 1997).

Kesey, Ken. *One Flew Over the Cuckoo's Nest* (New York: The Viking Press, 1962).

Killen, Andreas. *Berlin Electropolis: Shock, Nerves, and German Modernity* (Berkeley: University of California Press, 2006).

Klein, Naomi. *The Shock Doctrine: The Rise of Disaster Capitalism* (New York: Henry Holt and Company, 2007).

Kline, Wendy. *Bodies of Knowledge: Sexuality: Reproduction, and Women's Health in the Second Wave* (Chicago: University of Chicago Press, 2010).

Kneeland, Timothy W. and Carol A. B. Warren, *Pushbutton Psychiatry: A History of Electroshock in America* (Westport: Praeger Publishers, 2002).

Krim, Seymour. ed. *The Beats: A Gold Medal Anthology* (Greenwich, CT: Fawcett Publications, Inc., 1960).

Kruger, Judith. *My Fight for Sanity* (Greenwich: Crest Books, 1959).

Kukil, Karen V. ed. *The Unabridged Journals of Sylvia Plath, 1950–1962* (New York: Anchor Plath, Books, 2000).

Lakoff, Andrew. *Pharmaceutical Reason: Knowledge and Value in Global Psychiatry* (Cambridge: Cambridge University Press, 2005).

Laqueur, Thomas. *Making Sex: Body and Gender from the Greeks to Freud* (Cambridge: Harvard University Press, 1990).

Lederer, Susan. *Frankenstein: Penetrating the Secrets of Nature* (New Brunswick: Rutgers University Press, 2002).

Lisanby, Sarah H. ed. *Brain Stimulation in Psychiatric Treatment* (Washington, D.C.: American Psychiatric Publishing, Inc., 2004).

Lynn, Kenneth S. *Hemingway* (Cambridge: Harvard University Press, 1987) 578–579.

Malitz, Sydney and Harold A. Sackeim eds., *Electroconvulsive Therapy: Clinical and Basic Research Issues, Annals of the New York Academy of Sciences* (New York: The New York Academy of Sciences, 1986).

Manning, Martha. *Undercurrents: A Life beneath the Surface* (New York: HarperSanFrancisco, 1994).

Marks, Harry. *The Progress of Experiment: Science and Therapeutic Reform in the United States, 1900–1990* (Cambridge: Cambridge University Press, 1997).

Marks, John. *The Search for the Manchurian Candidate: The CIA and Mind Control* (New York: W. W. Norton and Company, 1979).

Martin, Emily. *The Woman in the Body: A Cultural Analysis of Reproduction* (Boston: Beacon Press, 1987).

———. *Bipolar Expeditions: Mania and Depression in American Culture* (Princeton: Princeton University Press, 2009).

McNeil, Legs and Gillian McCain, *Please Kill Me: The Uncensored Oral History of Punk* (New York: Penguin, 1996).

Menninger, Roy W. and John C. Nemaha eds., *American Psychiatry after World War II, 1944–1994* (Washington, D.C.: American Psychiatric Press, 2000).

Metzl, Jonathan. *Prozac on the Couch: Prescribing Gender in the Era of Wonder Drugs* (Durham, NC: Duke University Press, 2003).

———. *The Protest Psychosis: How Schizophrenia Became a Black Disease* (Boston: Beacon Press, 2009).

Micale, Mark S. and Roy Porter eds., *Discovering the History of Psychiatry* (Oxford: Oxford University Press, 1994).

Milner, Marion. *The Hands of the Living God: An Account of a Psycho-analytic Treatment* (London: Virago Press, 1988, originally published 1969).

Morus, Iwan Rhys. *Shocking Bodies: Life, Death, and Electricity in Victorian England* (Gloucestershire: The History Press, 2011).

Mosse, Eric P. *The Conquest of Loneliness* (New York: Random House, 1957).

Nasar, Sylvia. *A Beautiful Mind: The Life of Mathematical Genius and Nobel Laureate John Nash* (New York: Touchstone, 1998).

Nisbet, Robert. *Social Change and History: Aspects of the Western Theory of Development* (London: Oxford University Press, 1969).

Nuland, Sherwin. *Lost in America: A Journey with My Father* (New York: Alfred A. Knopf, 2003).

Nye, David. *Electrifying America: Social Meanings of a New Technology* (Cambridge: MIT Press, 1992).

Parsons, Talcott. *The Social System* (Glencoe: The Free Press, 1951).

Payer, Lynn. *Medicine and Culture* (New York: Penguin Books, 1988).

Perry, Helen Swick. *Psychiatrist of America: The Life of Harry Stack Sullivan* (Cambridge: The Belknap Press of Harvard University Press, 1982).

Pirsig, Robert M. *Zen and the Art of Motorcycle Maintenance: An Inquiry into Values* (New York: Bantam Books, 1974).

Plath, Sylvia. *The Bell Jar* (New York: Bantam Books, 1971, originally published 1963).

Popenoe, Paul. *Marriage Is What You Make It* (New York: The MacMillan Company, 1950).

Porter, Roy. *The Faber Book of Madness* (London: Faber and Faber, 1991).

Pressman, Jack D. *Last Resort: Psychosurgery and the Limits of Medicine* (Cambridge: Cambridge University Press, 1998).

Rabinbach, Anson. *The Human Motor: Energy, Fatigue, and the Origins of Modernity* (Berkeley: University of California Press, 1992).

Rasmussen, Nicolas. *On Speed: The Many Lives of Amphetamine* (New York: New York University Press, 2008).

Raz, Mical. *The Lobotomy Letters: The Making of American Psychosurgery* (Rochester: University of Rochester Press, 2013).

Reaume, Geoffrey. *Remembrance of Patients Past: Patient Life at the Toronto Hospital for the Insane, 1870–1940* (Oxford: Oxford University Press, 2000).

Reiser, Stanley Joel. *Medicine and the Reign of Technology* (Cambridge: Cambridge University Press, 1981).

Reverby, Susan and David Rosner, *Health Care in America: Essays in Social History* (Philadelphia: Temple University Press, 1979).

Ricoeur, Paul. *Time and Narrative* (Kathleen McLaughlin and David Pellauer, trans., Chicago: University of Chicago Press, 1984).

Rieff, Philip. *The Triumph of the Therapeutic: Uses of Faith after Freud* (Chicago: University of Chicago Press, 1966).

Rosenberg, Charles. *The Cholera Years: The United States in 1832, 1849, and 1866* (2nd edition, Chicago: University of Chicago Press, 1987).

Rowbottom, Margaret and Charles Susskind, *Electricity and Medicine: History of Their Interaction* (San Francisco: San Francisco Press, 1984).

Sadowsky, Jonathan. *Imperial Bedlam: Institutions of Madness and Colonialism in Southwest Nigeria* (Berkeley: University of California Press, 1999).

Saks, Elyn. *The Center Cannot Hold: My Journey through Madness* (New York: Hachette Books, 2007).

Scheff, Thomas. *Being Mentally Ill: A Sociological Theory* (2nd edition, Chicago: Aldine de Gruyter, 1982).

Scull, Andrew. *Madness in Civilization: A Cultural History of Schizophrenia from the Bible to Freud, from the Madhouse to Modern Medicine* (Princeton: Princeton University Press, 2015).

Shelley, Mary. *Frankenstein, or the Modern Prometheus* (New York: Signet Classic, 1965, originally published 1816).

Shephard, Ben. *A War of Nerves: Soldiers and Psychiatrists in the Twentieth Century* (Cambridge: Harvard University Press, 2001).

Shorter, Edward. *A History of Psychiatry: From the Era of the Asylum to the Age of Prozac* (New York: John Wiley & Sons, 1997).

———. *A Historical Dictionary of Psychiatry* (Oxford: Oxford University Press, 2005).

Shorter, Edward and David Healy, *Shock Therapy: A History of Electroconvulsive Treatment in Mental Illness* (New Brunswick: Rutgers University Press, 2007).

Showalter, Elaine. *The Female Malady* (New York: Viking, 1985).

Söderqvist, Thomas. ed. *The History and Poetics of Scientific Biography* (Burlington: Ashgate, 2007).

Solomon, Andrew. *The Noonday Demon: An Atlas of Depression* (New York: Scribner, 2001).

Starr, Paul. *The Social Transformation of American Medicine* (New York: Basic Books, 1984).

Staub, Michael E. *Madness Is Civilization: When the Diagnosis Was Social, 1948–1980* (Chicago: University of Chicago Press, 2011).

Steinfeld, Julius I. *Therapeutic Studies on Psychotics: A Psychological and Psychosomatic Approach in Four Papers* (Des Plaines, IL: Forest Press Publishers, 1951).

Sullivan, Harry Stack. *Conceptions of Modern Psychiatry* (Washington, D.C.: The William Alanson White Psychiatric Foundation, 1947).

Sulloway, Frank. *Freud: Biologist of the Mind* (New York: Basic Books, 1979).

Szasz, Thomas. *The Myth of Mental Illness: Foundations of a Theory of Personal Conduct* (New York: Harper Perennial, 2010, originally published 1961).

———. *The Manufacture of Madness: A Comparative Study of the Inquisition and the Mental Health Movement* (New York: Harper Torchbooks, 1970).

———. *Coercion as Cure: A Critical History of Psychiatry* (New Brunswick, NJ: Transaction Publishers, 2009).

Talland, George A. and Nancy C. Waugh eds., *The Pathology of Memory* (New York: Academic Press, 1969).

Tanner, Stephen L. *Ken Kesey* (Boston: Twayne Publishers, 1983).

Terry, Jennifer. *An American Obsession: Science, Medicine, and Homosexuality in Modern Society* (Chicago: University of Chicago Press, 1999).

Thomas, Gordon. *Journey into Madness: The True Story of Secret CIA Mind Control and Medical Abuse* (New York: Bantam Book, 1989).

Thompson, E. P. *The Making of the English Working Class* (New York: Vintage Books, 1966, originally published 1963).

Tomes, Nancy. *The Gospel of Germs: Men, Women, and the Microbe in American Life* (Cambridge: Harvard University Press, 1998).

Tone, Andrea. *The Age of Anxiety: America's Turbulent Affair with Tranquilizers* (New York: Basic Books, 2008).

Tone, Andrea and Elizabeth Siegel Watkins eds., *Medicating Modern America* (New York: New York University Press, 2007).

Tracy, Sarah W. *Alcoholism in America: From Reconstruction to Prohibition* (Baltimore: The Johns Hopkins University Press, 2005).

Valenstein, Elliot S. *Great and Desperate Cures: The Rise and Decline of Psychosurgery and Other Radical Treatments for Mental Illness* (New York: Basic Books, 1986).

Vogel, Morris J. and Charles E. Rosenberg eds., *The Therapeutic Revolution: Essays in the Social History of American Medicine* (Philadelphia: University of Pennsylvania Press, 1979).

Vonnegut, Mark. *The Eden Express* (New York: Bantam Books, 1976).

———. *Just like Someone without a Mental Illness, Only More So* (New York: Delacorte Press, 2010).

Ward, Mary Jane. *The Snake Pit* (Cutchogue, NY: Buccaneer Books, 1983, originally published 1946).

Warner, John Harley. *The Therapeutic Perspective: Medical Practice, Knowledge, and Identity in America, 1820–1885* (Princeton: Princeton University Press, 1997, originally published 1986).

Weinstein, Harvey. *A Father, A Son, and the CIA* (Toronto: James Lorimer and Company, 1988).

Whitty, C. W. M. and O. L. Zangwill, *Amnesia* (London: Butterworths, 1966).

Wolfe, Audra. *Competing with the Soviets: Science, Technology, and the State in Cold War America* (Baltimore: The Johns Hopkins University Press, 2013).

Wolfe, Ellen. *Aftershock: The Story of a Psychotic Episode* (New York: G. P. Putnam's and Sons, 1969).

Wortis, Joseph. ed. *Recent Advances in Biological Psychiatry* (New York: Plenum Press, 1968).

Zubin, Joseph and Howard F. Hunt eds., *Comparative Psychopathology: Animal and Human* (New York: Grune & Stratton, 1967).

Index